The 5 Day
Owner's Manual

Find your weight loss surgery tool in five focused days.

By Kaye Bailey

A LivingAfterWLS Publication

The 5 Day Pouch Test Owner's Manual

Find your weight loss surgery tool in five focused days.

Have you lost confidence in your weight loss surgery tool?

Welcome to the 5 Day Pouch Test. I am Kaye Bailey and I developed the 5 Day Pouch Test in 2007 through extensive research and personal experience. Seven years after gastric bypass I started to regain weight. Weight loss surgery became another diet failure, another disappointment. My surgeon told me to "get back to basics" but he didn't tell me how. Like most bariatric patients who see weight regain, I was on my own to figure it out or surrender one more time to obesity. No matter how I vowed each morning that this would be the day I quit snacking on the soft comfortable simple carbohydrates and get back to the weight loss surgery high protein diet, by noon I was dipping into the cracker barrel or popcorn bucket or cookie jar. The cycle of morning resolve followed by mid-day submission to cravings led to self-loathing and feelings of weakness and failure.

Have you found yourself in a similar cycle? Many of us do, but it's not because we are weak or spineless or moral failures. It turns out the human body's metabolic system is far stronger than willpower. I wasn't craving soft carbs by noon because I was morally weak. Those cravings were the body's "tune engine" alarm sounding too loudly to ignore. This knowledge powered the creation of the 5 Day Pouch Test where over the course of five days we do some engine maintenance and gently transition the body from simple carbs and snacks to the WLS high protein diet supported with complex carbohydrates found in vegetables, fruit, and grains.

The plan works because when we manage our metabolic system with the same attention we give to willpower there is nothing that can stop us.

If this scenario is familiar to you I invite you to give the 5 Day Pouch Test a try. If you make your plan today and follow Day 1 tomorrow by next week you will know how magnificent and powerful, you are. You own your WLS, and of course we all know WLS is "only a tool." Give the 5 Day Pouch Test a try. I bet you learn your tool is not broken; it just needs a little tune-up.

Thousands of people around the world have taken control of their surgical pouch by following the 5 Day Pouch Test. At the end of Day 5 many who were sad and hopeless at the beginning of the week report euphoria knowing the pouch is functioning properly. Hopelessness is replaced with confidence.

Five days. That is all it takes to turn things around.

A Few Good Words about the 5DPT:

"An exceptional resource for anyone who has had WLS. Very informative and written in a touching, humorous and gentle way. The recipes are excellent too." ~James M.S., Amazon Review October 13, 2015

"I have this book and live by it. Kaye Bailey is an advocate for those of us that have had weight loss surgery. She has written this book with love and experience. When I get off track from weight loss surgery and feel hopeless, I pick up this book and follow the 5 Day Pouch Test. In those five days I feel back in control and empowered. Another plus to doing the 5 Day Pouch Test is that I usually lose a few pounds as a bonus. I highly recommend this book to anyone who has had WLS. I have bought several of these books as gifts for my new WLS friends." ~Karen Gomes ~ September 4, 2013

"For those of you who have had Bariatric surgery this is a great book. If you ever get off track, the 5 Day Pouch Test will get you going again. Its detailed approach brings you back to the days after surgery and you can lose a few pounds. It really works." ~Kathleen S. Amazon Review, May 11, 2015

"This book is filled with ideas for recipes to help WLS patients keep on track with healthy eating. The book really helps because sometimes you just can't think of new ideas for meals. Kaye Bailey has an endless supply of great meal ideas that are easy and tasty." ~S.W. Amazon Review ~ May 8, 2015

"I have found the 5DPT to be invaluable. I regained my focus on this plan. Protein did feel uncomfortable so sliders were easier but until this plan I had not recognized this. Now I am on track and more importantly feel empowered and happy." ~Trudy S. Facebook, December 2014

Table of Contents

Thank you for joining me in the 5 Day Pouch Test program and making it a valued tool in your weight loss surgery toolbox. In your hands is the second edition of the 5 Day Pouch Test Owner's Manual. The original manual, first published in 2008 and reprinted several times since, has been updated with new FDA nutrition guidelines, updated policy from the bariatric field, and new studies relating to the treatment of obesity. You will also discover 16 new, tested and approved recipes included for your enjoyment during the 5 Day Pouch Test. In response to helpful feedback from readers of the first edition the format has been changed slightly making it easier to find quick answers while also providing complete discussions about the what, how, and why of working our weight loss surgery tool.

Chapters 1 and 2 introduce me and my experience to you and share how it is that we get to a place of weight regain after weight loss surgery. These chapters set the tone of personal empowerment, compassion, and kindness that you will find throughout the manual.

Chapter 3 is a brief overview of the 5 Day Pouch Test. A quick read here gives you a starting point for the plan, a quick review of the weight loss surgery Four Rules and tenets of successful weight management.

Moving on to Chapters 4, 5, and 6 each day is covered in detail. Chapters for each day include the dietary plan for the day, helpful and motivational sub-chapters, a summary of key learning points, one-page daily journal, and a series of Frequently Asked Questions specific to that day of the plan. These daily chapters should be reviewed frequently during the 5DPT to solidify your learning experience and help you transition to a Day 6 lifestyle of weight management.

Chapter 8 is a collection of miscellaneous questions about the 5 Day Pouch Test that are not specific any particular day of the plan. Please take a quick look, perhaps one of these questions is on your mind.

Chapter 9 takes us through a more comprehensive look at the Four Rules and other dietary basics of weight loss surgery. This is information we need to know and use as we work with our surgery to lose weight and keep it off. Please keep this reference in mind down the road if things are not going as planned. You just may find a nugget of information here that is helpful in getting you back on track. Even after a decade of living with weight loss surgery I still need reminders about what works with this wonderfully peculiar gastric system of mine. If you are prone to dumping syndrome be sure to have someone close to you read the sub-chapter emergency first aid for dumping syndrome: the information may come in handy one day.

The final text chapter, Chapter 10, takes a look beyond the 5 Day Pouch Test to what I call Day 6. Pulling from my 5DPT follow-up book, "Day 6: Beyond the 5 Day Pouch Test" we look at how we can continue working with our surgical tool to sustain long-term weight loss and health management with surgery.

Please consider this manual a workbook more than a textbook. Space is provided for notes so that you may become as much an author of this tool as I am. Mark you favorite passages and fold the page corners. You are the owner of this manual and your tool: you are empowered by this knowledge. Make it work for you.

Finally, the recipes to support the 5 Day Pouch Test are gathered and organized by day beginning on page 119. These tested recipes are proven effective when used as part of the 5DPT plan. Many of the recipes are so good you will continue to prepare and enjoy them well beyond the 5 Day Pouch Test.

The end pages include reference notes and tools and the index to help you quickly find what you are looking for

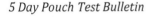

5 Day Pouch Test Bulletin

To receive our free monthly electronic newsletter, the "5 Day Pouch Test Bulletin", snap on the tag or visit 5DayPouchTest.com and enter your email address to subscribe. Also subscribe to our weekly "LivingAfterWLS Digest" and twice-monthly recipe newsletter, "Cooking with Kaye." We value and respect your online information: click the "Privacy" link on any of our web pages to learn more.

INTRODUCTION

Have you lost control of your weight loss surgery tool?

Does my pouch still work?

Have I broken my pouch?

Am I doomed to be a failure at this too?

Can I lose the weight I've regained?

Is the honeymoon period over?

I never made it to goal weight and now I'm gaining. Help!

If you are asking these questions, then the 5 Day Pouch Test is for you. In 5 focused days you can rediscover your pouch, get back on track and lose weight with your weight loss surgery tool. You have not failed. You can learn to use the tool again.

This is the five day plan that I developed and use to determine if my pouch is working and return to that tight newbie feeling. And a bonus to this plan: it helps one get back to the basics of the weight loss surgery diet and in most cases it triggers weight loss. It is not difficult to follow and if you are in a stage of snacking and carb-cycling it will break this pattern. Sounds pretty good, right?

The 5 Day Pouch Test should never leave you feeling hungry. You can eat as much of the prescribed menu foods as you want during the day to satiate hunger and prevent snacking on slider foods and white carbs. You must drink a minimum of 64 ounces of water each day. The liquid restrictions (no liquids 30 minutes before or after meals and no liquid with meals) must be observed.

5DPT = 5 Day Pouch Test

Weight loss is not the exclusive intent of the 5 Day Pouch Test. However, many who have completed this plan report a pleasing drop in weight. More importantly they celebrate a renewed sense of control over their pouch and eating habits. They easily transition back to a healthy post-surgical weight loss way of eating focused on lean-clean protein, vegetables, fruit, and limited dairy.

Countless thousands of people worldwide have successfully used the 5 Day Pouch Test since 2007 to take control of their weight loss surgery tool. Many have lost regained weight and others are reaching a healthy weight after long stalls in weight loss. But more importantly, feelings of failure are replaced with feelings of empowerment, capability, and personal achievement. Connect with others who have found the power of their pouch again with the 5DPT: Go to LivingAfterWLS.com and click on Neighborhood. I look forward to seeing you there and learning your story.

Push yourself as hard as you can in pursuit of your dreams.

Do you remember the 1970's best-selling book, Jonathan Livingston Seagull, by Richard Bach? The story is an allegory with a profound message.

Bach introduces us to Jonathan and his friend Fletcher, two seagulls that become impassioned to better themselves. They were not content to merely eat and sleep as seagulls do. They wanted to become extraordinarily good at what else they could do: fly. I often compare surgical weight loss patients to this classic story of two birds determined to become the very best at what they could do: fly. You, my friend, have the ability to become impassioned. You can soar. You can fly.

The 5 Day Pouch Test will give you the passion and wisdom.

Finally, you never have to walk alone in this journey. Online you will find knowledgeable, compassionate, and genuine support at the LivingAfterWLS Neighborhood. Local groups, sponsored by bariatric centers or individuals, are a valuable resource. Carefully selected family members, friends, and coworkers often provide motivation and encouragement. Reach out for whatever support system you are most comfortable with and empower one another. I believe in you, and I know you believe in me. We are a close-knit circle of friends. Together we can soar. Come on! Let's soar.

We are all in this together.
Kaye Bailey
KayeBailey@LivingAfterWLS.com

Our human evolution shows that our social connections are as essential to life as are food and water. We need one another to lean upon and to learn from and to lend support. Every human culture on Earth has a social structure through which the group connects for its very survival. In this age of electronic social media we are forming new social structures where people are brought together by similar experiences, beliefs, and goals. Through the Internet weight loss surgery patients from around the world have connected in the LivingAfterWLS Neighborhood *(now shuttered, see page 179)*, on the major social media sites, and other WLS-specific online communities. We never have to travel this path alone without the benefit and knowledge of others who understand. So let's connect. We are all in this together!

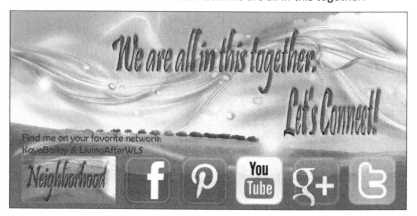

Facebook
http://www.facebook.com/LivingAfterWLS
Pinterest
http://pinterest.com/kayebaileylawls/
YouTube
http://www.youtube.com/user/KayeBailey
Google+
https://plus.google.com - Search Kaye Bailey
Twitter
https://twitter.com/LivingAfterWLS
Email:
KayeBailey@LivingAfterWLS.com

Chapter 1: Treat yourself kindly

This weight loss surgery is serious business.

Like so many others who ultimately undergo weight loss surgery, I battled obesity most of my life. It was on the first day of kindergarten I learned the three-letter word: fat. I did not know the word *fat* would define me for the rest of my life. I did not know what *fat* was; but I knew the little girl sitting next to me told me I was *fat* and I understood at once *fat* was a bad thing to be. Life would teach me that often people see fat first, and sometimes they do not look beyond the fat to see a person.

My work in the weight loss surgery community tells me you may share a similar story.

When I was growing up, obesity was considered a shameful personal flaw, not a disease. I watched my mom and my aunts; most of them overweight or morbidly obese, diet up and down the scale, chasing the latest fad-to-thinness, enjoying momentary success only to bounce right back up the scale. As a teenager I joined the yo-yo diet club and mirrored my examples losing and gaining time and time again. I entered college a full-figure size 18: I was one of the smiling sad fat girls.

Several years and many diets later I was not overweight: I was morbidly obese. With that comes shame, feelings of failure and self-loathing not to mention poor health and a sedentary lifestyle.

In the late 1990's there was buzz in the medical treatment of obesity about a new gastric surgery that was minimally invasive and highly effective. I knew about the primitive stomach stapling back in the 1980's and was fascinated by the weight loss transformation it caused. I wanted that transformation and finally felt I deserved it. With high hopes I underwent laparoscopic gastric bypass in September 1999.

Perhaps you, like me, sat through the pre-surgical counseling with your surgeon who looked you in the eye and said, *"Weight loss surgery is only a tool."* How many times have we heard that? It's only a tool. I nodded my head believing I understood what *"only a tool"* meant. Quite frankly, I had no clue what it meant. Secretly I hoped that surgery was, after all, going to be **"my easy way out."**

Weight loss was easy for me, *at first*. I was fortunate to have no complications and the weight came off quickly: I reached goal weight in the first year. Now, I do need to say I started a formal exercise program 14 days after surgery, and I was extremely compliant with the dietary guidelines; I was a model patient driven by the greatest determination I had ever known. I followed the Four Rules as if they were commandments.

The transformation was profound. Not only had I shed 130 pounds, I had shed that downtrodden self-loathing person for a new healthy confident trim woman. I held that weight for three years and I thrived.

But like so many others, a little bit here, a little bit there, and the weight started coming back. Perhaps I was careless with my food choices, or perhaps I was rebellious against the surgery and the pouch. Maybe there was too much celebrating, too much stress, too much to do, and no time to take care of myself. I ignored a five-pound gain. It was only five pounds, right? I quit visiting the bathroom scale, and I ignored the tightening feel of my clothing. Soon the five-pound gain was 30 pounds.

I was embarrassed, angry, and felt totally, hopelessly out of control. The old wicked diet pattern of losing and gaining, the very pattern that I believed surgery would cure, was back in my life. I could not believe I had become one of the many who gained weight back after surgery. How did this happen to me? How did I become one of *those* people? It is one thing to regain weight after losing on a mainstream diet: everyone expects regain after conventional weight loss, after all diets don't work, right? But a regain of weight after *"taking the easy way out"* with surgery is devastating.

Losing the edge; forgetting the promises.

If you have undergone a bariatric surgical procedure to control the metabolic disorder causing you to suffer from morbid obesity, then you understand what it means to jump through hoops. Unlike any other life threatening illness people suffering from morbid obesity must prove they are sick enough to undergo surgical intervention and at the same time demonstrate they are mentally healthy enough to adapt to that treatment and its consequences.

Like all WLS patients, I jumped through the hoops to get treatment with hell-bent determination that if I could just get this one break, some help from the good doctor, I would comply with the rules. I would never be *"one of those people"* who get the surgery only to briefly lose weight and gain it all back. I did everything in my power to convince myself, my doctors, my insurance company, and even my Lord that I would die a miserable sickly death of co-morbidities if I did not have surgery to lose weight and save my life.

And that hell-bent determination carried me well, *for a time.* I did lose weight and I did comply with the rules and restrictions of surgery. And I did praise my surgeon, and my insurance company, and my Lord that my life was spared and I was healthy, alive, and living. I suppose with all that praising going on I kind of lost sight of the path, left the course really, all in the name of *living.* Pretty soon I wasn't eating protein first or drinking lots of water. My daily exercise was hit-and-miss and a little snacking never hurt anyone, right? Somewhere the fighting survivor personality gave way to a what-me-worry wanderlust personality that didn't bother to follow the directions.

This learned: We cannot successfully manage our health with this surgery if we enable split-personality behavior.

The minute we give up the hell-bent fighter and survivor personality in exchange for the happen-chance dieter of lost-pounds-past we are at risk of gaining weight, of feelings of failure, and worst of all: we are at risk of succumbing to the metabolic disorder we fought so passionately to have treated with bariatric surgery. We cannot have it both ways. If we truly

"Our nation stands at a crossroads. Today's epidemic of overweight and obesity threatens the historic progress we have made in increasing American's quality and years of healthy life. Two-thirds of adults and nearly one in three children are overweight or obese. The sobering impact of these numbers is reflected in the nation's concurrent epidemics of diabetes, heart disease, and other chronic diseases. If we do not reverse these trends, researchers warn that many of our children—our most precious resource—will be seriously afflicted in early adulthood with medical conditions such as diabetes and heart disease. This future is unacceptable."

Regina M. Benjamin
US Surgeon General
January 2010

believe our obesity is a medical condition -*and by medical definition it is-* then we must yesterday, today, and forever consider it a medical condition. We cannot be gut-whacked one day for the sake of saving our life and the next day abandon the dietary rules like we could a few weight loss programs back when on a whim we joined a strip mall diet program advertising *"Guaranteed weight loss! Join Now! Walk-ins Welcome."*

"Obesity is a chronic, debilitating and potentially fatal disease."
American College of Gastroenterology – 2008

You see, this bariatric surgery, it is serious business.

There is no whimsy in the decision to get gut-whacked, no neon sign blinking "Walk-ins Welcome." No lose 10 pounds or get your money back promotion. This is surgery of the highest medical order[1].

Think back to the days and weeks prior to your surgery. Like me, you talked the subject to wearisome repetition with your closest confidant. You put your personal and financial affairs in order. You signed a liability release praying not to be the rare death-on-the-table, a risk to one in every one-hundred of us. You set goals. You made your expectations known: what you expected of yourself and what you expected from others as you sought their support in this last effort at saving your life from a slow painful death from the complications of morbid obesity. Your claims were heartfelt, sincere, and emphatic: You wanted to be there to see your children grown and maybe grandchildren too. You wanted to live.

Perhaps we don't remember how bad obesity felt.

It is a funny thing, the way the mind works. The healthier we become the less we remember how truly sick we were before surgery and before weight loss. Similar to the memory of pain reported following childbirth, findings indicate that the more positive our experience is with weight loss, the less vividly we recall the pain (physical and emotional) of obesity prior to weight loss. This suggests that when we fall off the wagon of dietary compliance it is not so

---

[1] "Of the many treatment approaches for obesity and its complications, bariatric surgery shows the most promise in achieving significant and sustained weight loss and resolution of associated metabolic comorbidities, when compared to combinations of medications, dietary, and behavioral modifications." (Barham K. Abu Dayyeh, 2011)

much about a moral breakdown or relenting to environmental pressure (think food pushers), but perhaps we simply don't remember how bad obesity felt. The same is likely true for a recovering addict who returns to the drug of choice: they simply do not recall the agony of the addiction. This could explain why highly intelligent people often repeat the cycle of recovery and relapse befuddling those around them. *Perhaps we simply don't remember how bad obesity felt.*

Hot! Don't touch!

Toddlers are taught very quickly not to touch a hot stove. It only takes three little sharply spoken words, *"Hot! Don't touch!"* and one breach of the command and even the dimmest child learns not to touch the hot stove because doing so causes immediate pain. Behavior modification therapy works in a similar manner for adults. Some are taught to wear a rubber band on the wrist and when temptation for relapse occurs the band is snapped in a *"Hot! Don't touch!"* alert that danger looms.

The problem we encounter in the recovery from morbid obesity is that the environmental factors that feed our metabolic disorder don't burn when we touch them. Chocolate cake tastes good and macaroni and cheese feels comforting when we eat it. There is no sting from the snap of a rubber band, no burn from the heat of the stove.

When we had surgery most of us vowed we would never go back to the state of morbid obesity and illness that lead us to the operating room in the first place.

A 1972 love anthem recorded by Luther Ingram gave us those memorable cheating words, *"If loving you is wrong, then I don't want to be right."* Remember that classic? How easily it could be the theme song in our forever battle of the bulge.

I dare say the best *"Hot! Don't touch!"* snap for us comes when we understand the risk for split personality behavior following a bariatric surgery for weight loss. While it doesn't seem desirable to dwell upon the pain we suffered from our obesity it would serve us well not to forget it. Photos are a good reminder. I suggest not just the usual "before" picture, but how about a photo of your prescription medications or the CPAP breathing machine you had to wear at night, or the cane or walker you needed because your mobility was impaired? Those photo reminders will feel very much like a snap on the wrist and catapult your personality to being hell-bent on sustained recovery.

When we had surgery most of us vowed we would never go back to the state of morbid obesity and illness that lead us to the operating room in the first place.

I am me; I am not my disease.

An affirmation: I was born with the disease obesity and by the time I was out of college it had advanced to morbid obesity. At age 33 my disease was treated with gastric bypass surgery which affected a loss of weight that put my disease, morbid obesity, in remission. Three years later I suffered a relapse of my disease with a weight gain of 30 pounds. Through dietary and lifestyle compliance and following the rules prescribed by my bariatric surgeon, I was able to put my disease, obesity, back in remission. I will always have the disease of morbid obesity and I am fortunate that I was able, at a young age, to be treated with the best medically available option.

The Facts:

- Obesity is a disease.
- Weight loss puts the disease in remission.
- Weight gain puts the disease in relapse.
- As with most diseases, those who suffer obesity are responsible to make dietary and lifestyle changes that work in tandem with medical treatment to keep our disease in remission.
- Like most diseases, relapse occurs: obesity manifests relapse in weight gain.
- We are never limited in the number of times we can actively affect behaviors to put obesity in remission: we always have another chance.
- Most importantly, I am not the disease, I have the disease.

Regain Is Likely: It is generally believed that 80 percent of people who undergo weight loss surgery will experience weight regain (relapse) of 10-30 pounds depending upon initial weight loss. It is further believed that 20 percent of those will relapse to their former weight and possibly gain more as the disease of morbid obesity advances. This relapse can be the result of failed gastric surgery (the surgery was improperly performed or medical device failure); a non-compliant patient who does not evolve their eating and exercise habits; the active intestine becoming more efficient at absorbing calories; and potential stomach pouch stretch. New findings published in 2011 also suggest dilation of the stoma after Roux-en-Y gastric bypass contributes to weight regain after surgery.[2] Dr. Anita Courcoulas, chief of minimally invasive bariatric and general surgery at the University of Pittsburgh Medical Center said, "Regaining weight down the road is a common phenomenon for weight loss patients. These patients need to be educated and prepared for it if it happens."

> ***relapse***: *noun. recurrence of disease after apparent recovery.*
>
> ***remission***: *noun. abatement of signs and symptoms of disease.*

100% Conviction: It is my experience that 100% of patients who take to the operating table for the treatment of their disease say, "I'm not going to be one of *those* people who regain weight after surgery." You can bet the farm I said that! Imagine my embarrassment and shame when I did in fact become one of *those* people. At the time I didn't understand my disease had relapsed, in part because I had relaxed my newly evolved eating and exercise habits, but also because my body has a metabolic disorder that causes it to store excess body fat. I thought I gained weight because I was a failure at surgery. In truth it was the disease itself that made sustaining a body weight suggesting remission extremely difficult. Add that to my relaxed efforts in

---

[2] "Although many factors are likely to contribute to weight regain after bypass surgery (preoperative body mass index, nutritional habits, self-esteem, mental health, socioeconomic status, and fistula formation), bariatric surgeons have believed that progressive dilation of the gastrojejunal stoma after RYGB is also a cause." (Barham K. Abu Dayyeh, 2011)

following the post-surgery protocol and I gained weight. Of course I gained weight! What else could I have expected?

I failed AGAIN! I am not alone in my feelings of failure over weight regain. Dr. Courcoulas said, "These are people who feel that they have failed at everything they tried [for weight control] in their lives. If they feel that they are failing surgery, they're embarrassed and they don't want to come back for help." How sad for us. When a cancer patient suffers a relapse do they take it as a personal failure? I sure hope not. Popular media perpetuates the belief that weight gain equals failure. WLS celebrities are splashed across mainstream media and tabloids alike for weight regain. But a celebrity cancer survivor who suffers a relapse is lauded for their bravery. With a relapse in obesity the celebrity becomes the brunt of jokes for late night comedians. No wonder we don't want to become one of *those* people, but the statistics are not on our side. Sadly, most of us who regain weight after weight loss surgery will believe we failed and we will diminish our self-worth because of it.

I Am Not Obese. Since kindergarten I believed the word *fat* defined me and I actually thought that was who I was because *"You are fat"* and *"I am fat"* were constant phrases in my world. By about age 40 I finally figured out that I am not fat. I have obesity, a disease. Have you heard a heart attack patient say, "I am heart disease" or a leukemia patient say, "I am cancer"? Of course not! That would be absurd and we wouldn't allow it. So it goes for the obese: we are not the disease! We have a disease that is part of the whole person that makes us the wonderfully unique and powerful person we are. You are you. I am me. We are not the disease!

Relapse to Remission: Just like other diseases, obesity relapse can be put into remission. There is hope! As noted above there are (at least) four reasons for relapse including: failed gastric surgery; a non-compliant patient who does not evolve their eating and exercise habits; the active intestine becoming more efficient at absorbing calories; and potential stomach pouch stretch and/or stoma dilation. Keeping in mind that statistically weight regain is likely, that you are not a failure, and that you are not the disease, you can pragmatically go about mapping a plan to reverse relapse.

Be kind, for everyone you meet is fighting a hard battle.

~Plato

Now we understand how we arrived at a place of frustration, disappointment, and perhaps self-criticism when our weight management efforts with surgery didn't go exactly as planned. It is time to release those hopeless feelings because they no longer serve a purpose in this journey. Now is the time we begin to treat ourselves kindly. Practice kindness on yourself in the same nurturing way you treat your loved ones with kindness. You have acknowledged the problem. With the help of the 5 Day Pouch Test, you may take charge and again move your disease into remission. You are not alone. I have been in your shoes and I know the pain of failure when I lost hope and became one of *those* people.

The thing is: We are all one of those people.

We didn't ask for obesity and we didn't ask for the fight of a lifetime to keep it under control. Treat yourself kindly. Find your personal hell-bent determination. You already know how courageous and powerful you are: you learned that when you underwent bariatric surgery. The 5 Day Pouch Test will help you find that place again through the course of five days focused on your mental and physical wellness. Pull out your strength and reserves and let's do this together.

What you can do if weight regain happens.

Speak with your bariatric center. According to the American Society of Metabolic and Bariatric Surgeons[3] inadequate weight loss or weight regain should prompt evaluation for (1) surgical failure with loss of integrity of the gastric pouch in gastroplasty or RYGB (2) testing for enlarged GJ stoma diameter, (3) a poorly adjusted gastric band, and (4) development of maladaptive eating behaviors or psychological complications. (Jeffrey I. Mechanick, 2008).

Find a bariatric center on the official website for the American Society for Metabolic and Bariatric Surgeons. http://asmbs.org/

---

[3] The American Society for Metabolic and Bariatric Surgery (ASMBS) is the largest society for this specialty in the world. The vision of the Society is to improve public health and well-being by lessening the burden of the disease of obesity and related diseases throughout the world. http://asmbs.org/

Honest evaluation. Assess your eating and exercise evolution and return to the lifestyle prescribed at the time of surgery. Use the 5 Day Pouch Test as a mechanism for returning to dietary and lifestyle compliance prescribed at the time of surgery.

Pursue knowledge. Become educated on nutritional health, physical fitness, and spiritual wellness so they may work in harmony to heal your body. Act upon what you learn. Take action. Knowledge is a powerful tool in our pursuit of healthy weight management.

Enlist help. Seek the support of family, friends, community, health care professionals, and fellow patients to help maintain your personal investment and motivation. By the same token: give support. Empowering others is a dynamic exercise in personal motivation.

Weight regain is complicated. Remember, weight regain following weight loss surgery is not a simple matter. According to experts, "Weight regain after gastric surgery is multi-factorial and likely involves a complex interplay between a permissive psychosocial environment, nutritional habits, and a complex genetic and anatomic milieu that effect many physiological regulatory pathways controlling food intake behavior and energy metabolism after the procedure." (Barham K. Abu Dayyeh, 2011)

Chapter 2: Fixing broken windows

Surgery is only a tool.

There is a popular theory in urban renewal that suggests fixing broken windows as they happen is the key to reducing crime and preventing urban decay. George Kelling discusses the theory in a 1982 Atlantic Monthly article. He writes, "Consider a building with a few broken windows. If the windows are not repaired the tendency is for vandals to break a few more windows. Eventually, they may even break into the building, and if unoccupied, become squatters or cause destruction inside."

I believe it is possible to apply the *"Broken Window"* theory to our post-weight loss surgery health and wellness. The broken window, of course, would be a lapse in compliance with our program: eating unhealthy foods, the absence of exercise, and ignoring the rules. If we break a window one day and do not fix it the next then we risk breaking another window. But if we practice self-renewal and fix that broken window promptly we can avoid the intrusion of vandals and squatters who would break more windows and violate our bodies.

The challenge herein is that if we allow the broken window to go without repair we then become the vandals to our own body. At times it is far easier to give permission to the squatters than it is to evict them. One day of missed exercise leads to another and another and pretty soon the sloth-squatter has set-up camp in our building: our body. Over the holidays I missed several workout sessions and my sloth-squatter became quite at home enjoying free entry through my broken windows. When this happens immediate action must be taken to kick that squatter out. With determined self-renewal we must take control of our house.

Broken windows happen.

Broken windows happen. In our homes and in our lives there will always be broken windows. A broken window is not a sign of failure or neglect. Windows are made of fragile glass that sometimes shatters. And though we may pretend to be tough as steel we are more like glass: fragile and prone to occasional breakage. Windows can be fixed. Let's fix our broken windows promptly and forbid the squatter's entry. We have worked hard for our new life. We deserve the gift of self-renewal.

The 5 Day Pouch Test will teach you to fix your broken windows. This is a highly structured back-to-basics five day plan that effectively repairs our broken windows and reminds us of the rules and guidelines that helped us use our tool to lose weight with surgery in the first place. The exclusive intent is not to lose weight: it is to get back-to-basics. Now is the time to repair our broken windows.

The 5 Day Pouch Test is most successful when we prepare mentally and emotionally to follow the plan as written and emerge on Day 6 enthusiastic to follow the Four Rules, make healthy food choices, exercise, and live well. The empowered feeling you get from completing the 5 Day Pouch Test will fuel a mental storm of enthusiasm similar to the excitement and can-do feelings you enjoyed during the early phase of weight loss following your surgical procedure.

As we discussed in Chapter 1 it is imperative we find the hell-bent determination that led us to have weight loss surgery in the first place. We must actively recover the storm of enthusiasm that worked so well for us in the beginning of this experience. Think back when you were researching weight loss surgery: the sleepless nights imagining finally having a method of weight control that would work and you could get off the dieting roller coaster. This is the kind of determination we need in order to get back on track. Ayn Rand, the noted 20th century philosopher, wrote,

"The question isn't who is going to let me;
The question is who is going to stop me."

It is with this kind of hell-bent determination that we jumped through hoops to have the surgery. The same grit determination must be employed after surgery. If we are to achieve a healthy life we absolutely must fight like a mad dog against everything that made us obese in the first place. We must take control and own responsibility for our success.

Our highly skilled bariatric surgeons are giving us the best tool medically possible for the treatment of chronic obesity. Gastric banding, gastric sleeve, and gastric bypass are state of the art medically effective ways for treating obesity long-term. It is our responsibility to use this tool to the best of our ability combined with other tools including diet, exercise, mental reconditioning, mental toughness and ongoing support networks. Not only is this our responsibility: we deserve the healthy rewards that come when we maximize the potential of this tool.

You deserve to thrive in your best healthy life.

Surgery is only a tool.

Surgery is only a tool. A tool is simply a device used to accomplish a task. Think of a carpenter at the workbench with his tools. Before the carpenter: a saw, a hammer, wood, a measuring stick and nails: all tools of the trade. The carpenter could stand before the tools and yearn for them to craft a magnificent treasure box. But the tools will not work on yearning alone. The carpenter must select the best tool for the task and then work with that tool using it to the best of his capability. The carpenter must work the tools.

And so it goes with our weight loss surgery tool. Yearning and desire will not cause the tool to craft the treasure of a healthy body. The tool will not work on hope alone.

As owners of this powerful weight loss surgery tool we become stewards to work for it, to pursue our greatest potential through knowledge, practice, and personal responsibility.

A tool is simply a device used to accomplish a task. The tool will not work on hope alone. We must work the tool to the best of our capability.

We must use the tool as a device to accomplish a task. If the tool breaks, such as a band slippage or failure, we must go to the repair shop for maintenance. *The care of the tool is our responsibility.* When we take responsibility for working the tool our chances for lasting success are great.

If we get comfortable in our post-weight loss surgery life there is a tendency to lose our determination. Perhaps we take it for granted. Maybe we just get bored or distracted. Maybe we get discouraged because life after surgery has been a struggle. Any of these things can cause us to lose hope or feel like failures. I have gone through periods of sadness and periods of euphoria since my weight loss surgery. Haven't you?

But just like we can work a plan to test the pouch, and work the tools, we can mentally train our mind to get back to being hell-bent determined to take personal control of our health. The 5 Day Pouch Test is the second step back to control. You have already taken the first step: seeking help. That is why you are here.

Now is the time to identify where you went off track. You will not be judged or made fun of. We all fall off track now and again. Be kind to yourself. A broken window is not a moral breakdown or personal failure; it is the product of living. Fixing the broken window is your responsibility. I am your champion in this cause.

The Plan to Work the 5 Day Pouch Test.

It sounds silly to offer a plan to work a plan but here I present a few ideas and hints for making the most of your 5DPT experience. The more prepared and enthused you are when you begin the 5DPT, the better your chances for success. Let's get started and let's get back on track!

Learn the plan. Read the plan in full and be sure you understand it. Read the plan completely in order to understand the progression of your diet from Day 1 to Day 5. Pay close attention to understanding the liquid restrictions and slider foods: these are the most common problem areas that lead to weight regain after weight loss surgery. As you become familiar with the 5 Day Pouch Test think

Remember, you already know how to lose weight using your surgical tool.

back to how it compares with the early dietary stages following your weight loss surgery. Think back to what worked for you then and imagine the same will work for you again. Remember, you already know how to lose weight using your surgical tool. The effort you put into the 5DPT will return you to that place of healthy and reasonable weight management using your tool.

Mark the date. Set a date and mark your calendar. Make sure you can follow the plan without the disruption of travel, social events or hormonal cycles. Enlist the support of family and friends. It is fairly common for people to schedule the 5DPT to begin on Monday and end on Friday. But many have found that scheduling Day 1 for a Saturday works more favorably for them. On Days 1 and 2 one generally needs frequent bathroom breaks, which may be uncomfortable in a workplace. Consider that as you schedule your plan. Additionally, many of us have made the mistake of completing the 5DPT on Friday only to celebrate with weekend binge eating come Saturday. If our plan starts on Saturday and concludes on Wednesday we can more easily transition to a Day 6 lifestyle on Thursday, thus avoiding the weekend binge phenomenon. Consider all of this before scheduling your 5 Day Pouch Test. Scheduling it for the right time significantly improves our chance for success.

Seek peer support. Decide who you will include in your plan and make known your expectations. Post to the Neighborhood or your online community asking for support from those who understand. The correct peer support nurtures our efforts in this recovery from relapse. We can learn from those who have traveled this path and tap into their enthusiasm. It is the nature of online support communities to cheer and celebrate each other's victories as well as buoy those who are struggling. Take advantage of this and gather your own cheering section to celebrate the baby steps that become big accomplishments. Become a support peer to others; when we are in this together: support of one another is symbiotic.

We are all in this together!

Make preparations. Plan your meals for all five days and do the grocery shopping before starting the 5DPT. We all know that the supermarket is temptation alley, do your best to avoid going there for these five days. An effective way to plan your meals is to use the 5 Day Pouch Test menu plan in Chapter 3. Make two copies of the 5DPT menu plan and use the first to plan your meals and snacks for all five days. This will become your shopping list as well as your map for the week. Many people are surprised at the relief and empowerment they feel upon making their food plan for five days. With the menu choices made there is little to dwell upon and we have spare energy to focus on getting back on track. In addition to finding the 5DPT menu plan in this manual you can always download it free from the website. Please use this valuable tool.

5DayPouchTest.com – Click on Tools

Mental readiness. Devote time to meditation focused on the 5 Day Pouch Test: why you are doing it and what you wish to accomplish. You practiced mental readiness before surgery and it served you well. Do the same now. Practice the self-kindness we talked about in Chapter 1 and accept that windows get broken, then eagerly anticipate making repairs. You are about to embark on the repair process and exciting and good things will come to you for your initiative to take action. This is exciting stuff! Practice meditation your own way and build the excitement. If that means writing in a journal or listening to music or just spending quiet time thinking, then do it. Mental readiness is essential in every life-endeavor worth taking.

The night before Day 1 create a storm of mental readiness by reading, discussing, and imagining your personal power to work the plan. Generate the same kind of excitement you had going into surgery. Go to bed empowered knowing you are about take control of the surgical tool you fought so hard to get in the first place.

Take time to ponder the questions on the "I Can Do This" contract at the end of this chapter. Be true to yourself and be kind to yourself. Give yourself the same eager support and compassion you would give your best friend.

Please use the 5 Day Pouch Test as your vehicle of change.

Rise and Shine! Welcome to Day 1! Step on the scale and record your weight. Start Day 1 off right with your carefully planned meal and look forward to the next meal knowing you have already made the right food choice. Consider how happy your little gastric pouch is to be nurtured with gentle soft liquids; how good it feels to be healing from the cycle of poor food choices. Treating your body well is never a punishment, it is a gift to be enjoyed and celebrated. Please, allow yourself this.

*I was very sad to read this comment on an online forum; "I've done it (5DPT) several times and sure it helps for a week. Then the following week you are back to your normal cravings and even gain a pound or two." It is true that many who do the 5 Day Pouch Test with the mistaken intent to drop a few pounds quickly return to the same eating behavior they practiced before the 5DPT. As we have heard throughout our weight management lives: **If you continue to do the same thing you will continue to get the same results.** When the 5 Day Pouch Test is used correctly it gets us back on track in a manner that allows us to change course so that we might get different more desirable results.*

Over the next five days treat yourself kindly. As you see, kindness is a repeating theme in the 5 Day Pouch Test. The 5DPT isn't about perfection. It is a systematic method of breaking the slider carbohydrate cycle, returning to a weight loss surgery way of eating, and empowering you with the knowledge that your surgical tool works and *you can work the tool*. Nobody has ever done the 5DPT perfectly. But many have worked it well enough to find confidence and power in their tool.

Focus on the plan during the next five days. Stay enthused by connecting with others. Turn "Head-Hunger" into "Life Hunger". Nothing is more powerful than "Life Hunger" - the yearning for all the good things to be enjoyed when we release unhealthy eating and the self-loathing that accompanies it.

Use the 5 Day Pouch Test Journal to make a record of your experience. This tool is crucial in capturing the moment and making note of key learning experiences. Many scholars believe that we have a higher rate of memory retention when we record an experience in writing. This document will serve you well during the 5DPT and later down the road when you need a refresher of what you learned doing it. It only takes a few minutes each day to write on your journal, a small investment for the benefits it provides.

Keep learning. Use the 5 Day Pouch Test and beyond to continue your education about health, nutrition, weight management, and living after weight loss surgery. Continued education works to keep us informed, trying new things, and renewed hope that lasting remission from our medical disorder is achievable. Seek knowledge from reputable publications and from peers. This process of support and learning becomes a self-fulfilling prophecy as we benefit from the give-and-take of a generous spirit. Learn, teach, and share. We are in this together.

"Simply not wanting to be overweight is a wish, not a plan. One way to motivate yourself is to recognize how gratifying it is to make a commitment to a goal, identify the specific steps to get there, follow your plan, and reap the rewards." (Judith J. Wurtman & Nina Frusztajer Marquis, 2006)

Now that I have laid this out for you I want to bring back the pom-poms and the cheerful optimism. The surgical tool gives us something no strip-mall *"Walk-ins Welcome"* weight loss program ever will: the ability to bounce back time and time again. There is no limited quota on "do-overs" using our WLS tool. We can get back on track and we can work our stomach pouch to manage our metabolic disorder. We have learned how good it can feel to manage our weight and we can do it again. So harness that hell-bent personality. Grab your original goal by the love handles and take charge of your destiny. I am here for you and we are in this together. Not for just a few pounds; not just to goal weight. We are in this together for the purpose of *living*. You can do this! Ponder these questions as you make a personal contract with yourself:

It is best to act with confidence;
No matter how little right you have to it.
-Lillian Hellman

Do I have broken windows in my surgical weight loss house?

Do I wish to repair my broken windows at this time?

Do I deserve to fix my broken windows and enjoy the beauty of living a healthy and whole life?

How will I fix my broken windows and repair my surgical weight loss tool?

Do I have a plan I can follow and am I committed to that plan?

To whom will I be accountable?

Do I have a support system in place?

Am I prepared to treat myself kindly as I embark on a new chapter of living after weight loss surgery?

Am I head-hungry for living?

Chapter 3: The 5 Day Pouch Test plan

Find your tool in five focused days.

This chapter presents the nuts and bolts of the 5 Day Pouch Test. First the plan is briefly reviewed; use this overview as a quick reference throughout the five days to keep track of where you are and where you are going. Next are the basic tenets that apply to Days 1 through 5 and beyond the 5DPT. With a brief overview and the basics learned we now take a detailed look at each day of the 5DPT: the nitty-gritty of the plan. The days are organized in chapters: each includes the daily plan and supporting topics, key learning points, a daily journal and FAQ's pertinent to that day. You will find supporting recipes for each day of the 5DPT in the recipe section of this manual.

5DPT: Brief Overview.

It is only five days. And in the next five days you will learn your pouch is working; you will take control of your eating and snacking behaviors; and you will remember why you had weight loss surgery in the first place.

Days 1 and 2 of the plan are healing days. You treat your pouch like a newborn with gentle liquids and soups. Pouch inflammation is reduced and processed carbohydrate cravings subside. Mental focus is on listening to and respecting your body. Days 1 and 2 mimic the early days and weeks following bariatric surgery.

Day 3 introduces soft proteins like canned fish, fresh soft fish or eggs. This is the day we focus on tasting our food, chewing well, and enjoying the goodness of lean-clean protein. We focus on portion control and the liquid restrictions. On this day we start to remember what a tight pouch feels like and we appreciate the feeling of fullness.

Day 4 brings us to firm proteins like ground meat (beef, poultry, lamb, or game) and shellfish, scallops, lobster, salmon or halibut steaks. This is the day we truly realize the power of the pouch and most people are happily surprised to learn their pouch is not broken or stretched back to normal stomach size. The carbohydrate withdrawal is over, and energy levels are improving.

Day 5 finishes the test with solid proteins such as white meat poultry, beef steak, and any of the firm proteins from Day 4. The liquid restrictions are now a habit and we have successfully removed the slider foods from our diet. We have energy for exercise and for the daily tasks of living. Most importantly, we know our weight loss surgery tool works and we now have the confidence and capability to work the tool.

Day 6 is the way we will eat every day for the rest of our lives. Having successfully broken a carb-cycle, gained a feeling of control over the surgical gastric pouch, and possibly losing a few pounds one is ready for re-entry into a compliant way of eating. This means focusing on protein dense meals, observing the liquid restrictions, and avoiding starches, particularly processed carbohydrates and slider foods. Three meals a day should be two-thirds protein, one-third healthy carbohydrate in the form of low-glycemic vegetables and fruits. Consumption of whole grains is not forbidden, but should be limited to one serving a day.

Basic tenets applied during the 5DPT.

The following basic tenets are widely accepted by bariatric surgeons and nutritionists as lifestyle guidelines to be followed by people who have undergone all manner of gastric surgery for weight loss. I have found that making these tenets a lifestyle is the most effective way for me and many others to manage weight loss and maintain it with weight loss surgery. Refer to the documentation provided you at the time of your surgery for the specifics advised by your bariatric center. For our purposes each rule or tenet is summarized here for reference when learning and doing the 5 Day Pouch Test. Turn to Chapter 9, Dietary Basics of Weight Loss Surgery, to study in detail these principles and learn why they work. Always keep in mind that we are doing the 5DPT to correct behavior and change trajectory so we may achieve different and more desirable results.

Four Rules: Weight Loss Surgery basics

As patients we are well aware that WLS is frequently perceived by outsiders as an easy means to weight loss that requires little or no effort by the patient. It turns out there is nothing easy about the post-WLS lifestyle. At the time of surgery, we agreed to follow Four Rules of dietary and lifestyle management guidelines for the rest of our life in order to lose weight and maintain a healthy weight. This is our burden and our responsibility if we wish to keep morbid obesity in remission.

All surgical weight loss procedures including gastric bypass, adjustable gastric banding (lap-band) and gastric sleeve, promote weight loss by decreasing energy (caloric) intake with a reduced or restricted stomach size. The small stomach pouch is only effective when a patient rigorously follows the Four Rules: eat a high protein diet; drink lots of water; avoid snacking on empty calorie food; engage in daily exercise.

In our introduction to a bariatric program we were taught *and agreed* to follow the standard Four Rules which work in concert with our surgically altered stomach and digestive system to bring about rapid massive weight loss. In fact, most of us were asked during the psychological evaluation if we could commit to following the Four Rules. Like me, I bet you said "Of course" with complete confidence. What I missed in the orientation was that these rules would be a way of life for the *rest* of my life. The Four Rules and other WLS dietary basics are discussed in greater detail in Chapter 9. For now, let's take a quick look at each rule as it applies to WLS patients.

Protein First

Lots of Water

No Snacking

Daily Exercise

Protein First: At every meal the WLS patient will eat lean animal, dairy, or vegetable protein before any other food. Protein shakes or supplements may be included as part of the weight loss surgery diet. Patients are advised to consume 60-105 grams of protein a day. Eating lean protein will create a tight feeling in the surgical stomach pouch: this feeling is the signal to stop eating. Many patients report discomfort when eating lean protein, yet this discomfort is the very reason the stomach pouch is effective in reducing food and caloric intake. Animal products are the most nutrient rich source of protein and include fish, shellfish, poultry, and meat. Dairy protein, including eggs, yogurt, and cheese, is another excellent source of protein.

Lots of Water: Like most weight loss programs, bariatric surgery patients are instructed to drink lots of water throughout the day. Most centers advise a minimum of 64 fluid ounces of water each day. Water hydrates the organs and cells and facilitates the metabolic processes of human life. Water flushes toxins and waste from the body. Patients are strongly discouraged from drinking carbonated beverages. In addition, patients are warned against excessive alcohol intake as it tends to have a quicker and more profound intoxicating affect compared with pre-surgery consumption. In addition, non-nutritional beverages of any kind may lead to weight gain and increased snacking.

No Snacking: Patients are discouraged from snacking which may impede weight loss and lead to weight gain. Specifically, patients are forbidden to partake of traditional processed carbohydrate snacks, such as chips, crackers, baked goods, and sweets. Patients who return to snacking on empty calorie non-nutritional food defeat the restrictive nature of the surgery and weight gain results. It is seemingly contradictory that the 5DPT allows snacking. High protein snacks are allowed because they keep the metabolism active, they satiate hunger, and they help relieve the symptoms of carbohydrate withdrawal.

Daily Exercise: In general patients are advised to engage in 30 minutes of physical activity on most days of the week. The most effective way to heal the body from the ravages of obesity is to exercise. Exercise means moving the body: walking, stretching, bending, inhaling and exhaling. Exercise is the most effective, most enjoyable, most beneficial gift one can receive when recovering from life threatening, crippling morbid obesity. Consistent exercise will keep morbid obesity in remission and help compensate for lapses in following the three other rules. People who successfully maintain their weight exercise daily. In Chapter 9 we look at ways to make exercise fun and part of our activity of daily living.

Slider Foods & Liquid Restrictions

Slider Foods: To the weight loss surgery patient slider foods are the bane of good intentions often causing dumping syndrome, weight loss plateaus, and eventually weight gain. By definition slider foods are soft simple processed carbohydrates of little or no nutritional value that slide right through the surgical stomach pouch without providing nutrition or satiation. The most commonly consumed slider foods include pretzels, crackers (saltines, graham, Ritz®, etc.) filled cracker snacks such as Ritz Bits®, popcorn, cheese snacks (Cheetos®) or cheese crackers, tortilla chips with salsa, potato chips, sugar-free cookies, cakes, and candy.

The very nature of the surgical gastric pouch is to cause feelings of tightness or restriction when one has eaten enough food. However, when soft simple carbohydrates are eaten this tightness or restriction does not result and one can continue to eat, unmeasured amounts of food without ever feeling uncomfortable. Many patients unknowingly turn to slider foods for this very reason. They do not like the discomfort that results when the pouch is full from eating a measured portion of lean animal or dairy protein, and it is more comfortable to eat the soft slider foods. Slider foods have played a significant role in every case of post-WLS weight regain that I have ever heard about.

Liquid restrictions: After surgical weight loss patients are advised to avoid drinking liquids 30 minutes before meals and 30 minutes after meals. *(The time restriction varies from surgeon to surgeon, but most use the 30 minutes before, 30 minutes after restriction. Follow your surgeon's specific directions.)* In addition, there should be no liquid consumed while eating. Following these liquid restrictions allows the pouch to feel tight sooner and stay tight longer, thus leaving the patient feeling satiated for greater periods of time without experiencing the urge to snack. In addition, the longer food stays in the small gastric pouch the more opportunity the body has to absorb nutrients from that food. The liquid restrictions should be followed when eating all meals and snacks, including protein shakes, protein bars, hearty soups, and solid protein main dishes. Learn more in Chapter 9 about managing Rule 2 – *Lots of Water* - while observing the liquid restrictions.

Do you have a grumpy pouch? Here is a healing soup to ease your pouchy woes. Many times when we turn to the 5 Day Pouch Test we have been eating all the wrong things and we have an inflamed digestive system; sometimes we call this a grumpy pouch. If you are feeling particularly poorly going into the 5DPT consider making this soup the day before and enjoy the healing benefits of the ingredients that are natural digestive aids. This recipe is a great remedy any time you experience a grumpy pouch, use it even when you are not following the 5 Day Pouch Test.

Fennel and celery are both good digestive healers. Fennel is known to soothe an inflamed digestive lining and celery helps to support liver function. Raw vegetables can irritate an inflamed digestive system so this well-cooked soup soothes the digestive system and helps cleanse your body of toxins. Feel free to enjoy a 1-cup serving as a snack on any day of the 5DPT. Remember to observe the liquid restrictions, especially when eating soup. You want to make sure your body has time to absorb and digest the wholesome nutrients that come from a carefully made soup.

Fennel and Celery Soup

Ingredients:
1 large white or yellow onion, chopped (about 1 cup)
2 bulbs of root fennel, peeled and chopped
8 ribs of celery, chopped
4 cups vegetable stock, reduced-sodium
2 bay leaves
1 tablespoon fresh parsley, finely chopped
Parsley sprigs for garnish

Place all of the ingredients in a large saucepan and bring to a boil. Reduce to a low boil and cook for 10 minutes. Further reduce temperature to a slow simmer and cook an additional 30 minutes. Remove from heat and allow cooling. Remove and discard the bay leaves. Using a blender or immersion blender puree the soup until smooth. Return to saucepan and gently reheat. Thin the soup to desired consistency with additional vegetable broth. Enjoy a 1-cup serving of soup garnished with parsley sprigs. This soup keeps well refrigerated for three to four days. Serve gently reheated on the stovetop or in the microwave oven.

I have never done the 5DPT perfectly and I do not know anyone that has. Rather than make the five days about perfection make this time about learning. Little mistakes will not stop the world from turning. So forge ahead doing your very best and forgive little mistakes. Learn from each day, make notes on your 5 Day Pouch Test Journal, and emerge on Day 6 knowing more about yourself and how to work your tool. *You can do this!*

If we complete the 5 Day Pouch Test having learned a few things about our self, our weight loss surgery and our capability in managing life and weight loss surgery in relationship to one another we have succeeded: we can deem the 5 Day Pouch Test a success. Here are some things to consider while embracing the 5DPT as a learning experience:

- What can I eat that gives my pouch a feeling of fullness? What do I eat that fails to give my pouch a feeling of fullness?
- Have the liquid restrictions become automatic to me? Do I have heightened awareness of how I consume liquids with my meals and snacks?
- Am I eating protein in a ratio of 2 bites protein to 1 bite complex carbohydrate? (2B/1B Rhythm)
- Have I found time to include physical activity in my daily routine?
- Am I allowing myself to feel empowered when I make choices that nourish my body and respect my weight loss surgery?
- Am I forgiving lapses in compliance with my guidelines and moving forward to make better choices the next time?

One of the best ways to enable your success with the 5 Day Pouch Test is to plan in advance your meals for the duration of the plan. This is not a difficult task as you are only planning for five days. Many find having a complete plan to be liberating: the decision making is done. One must only concentrate on following the plan and focusing on surgical pouch and how it functions when used properly. Here are some helpful suggestions for planning your 5DPT menu:

For each day plan three meals (breakfast, lunch, dinner) and two or three snacks. Foods from Days 1 and 2 may be advanced to Days 3, 4, and 5. Do not bring foods from Days 3, 4, and 5 back to Days 1 and 2.

Purchase and store groceries for the 5DPT before Day 1 and avoid going to the market during the five days. The 5DPT will help build your resistance to marketing temptation, but during the five days the temptation may simply be an annoying distraction.

If you haven't tried protein gelatin or protein pudding before make a sample before your 5DPT. Make certain that what you plan is something you will enjoy eating. Consider 1-cup servings of soup as a suitable snack on any day of the 5DPT.

If including soups on Days 1 and 2 prepare them in advance before Day 1 and divide into 1-cup serving containers for ease of use.

All of the 5DPT recipes are healthy and family friendly. Try to include the people at your table in your menu and avoid cooking two meals. For others add vegetables, a salad or a starch as desired.

Try to stick with your menu plan as closely as possible. Sometimes change is unavoidable. Do the best you can at each meal staying as close to your plan as possible.

As always, practice kindness.

Day 1:
> Breakfast: Choco-Mocha Morning Smoothie
> Morning Snack: High-Protein Gelatin or 1 small orange
> Lunch: Vanilla-Berry Smoothie
> Afternoon Snack: 1/2 apple
> Dinner: 1 cup 5DPT soup of your Choice
> Evening Snack: High Protein Pudding

Day 2:
> Breakfast: Choco-Mocha Morning Smoothie
> Morning Snack: Frozen Protein Pudding Pop
> Lunch: 1 cup 5DPT soup of your choice
> Afternoon Snack: High Protein Gelatin
> Dinner: 1 cup 5DPT soup of your Choice
> Evening Snack: High Protein Pudding

Day 3:
> Breakfast: Mock Breakfast Burrito
> Morning Snack: High Protein Gelatin
> Lunch: Parmesan Tuna Patty
> Afternoon Snack: Frozen Protein Pudding Pop
> Dinner: Parmesan Tuna Patty
> Evening Snack: High Protein Gelatin

Day 4:
> Breakfast: Spinach-Sausage Egg Bake
> Morning Snack: 1 small orange
> Lunch: Parmesan Tuna Patty (leftover from Day 3)
> Afternoon Snack: 1 small pear and 1/2 cup cottage cheese
> Dinner: Orange Glazed Salmon
> Evening Snack: High Protein Pudding

Day 5:
> Breakfast: Egg Brunch Bake
> Morning Snack: 1 piece of low-glycemic fruit
> Lunch: Orange Glazed Salmon (leftover from Day 4)
> Afternoon Snack: High Protein Gelatin
> Dinner: Chicken and Pea Pods
> Evening Snack: Frozen Protein Pudding Pop

Day 1:
   Breakfast:

   Morning Snack:

   Lunch:

   Afternoon Snack:

   Dinner:

   Evening Snack:

Day 2:
   Breakfast:

   Morning Snack:

   Lunch:

   Afternoon Snack:

   Dinner:

   Evening Snack:

Day 3:
   Breakfast:

   Morning Snack:

   Lunch:

   Afternoon Snack:

   Dinner:

   Evening Snack:

Day 4:
   Breakfast:

   Morning Snack:

   Lunch:

   Afternoon Snack:

   Dinner:

   Evening Snack:

Day 5:
   Breakfast:

   Morning Snack:

   Lunch:

   Afternoon Snack:

   Dinner:

   Evening Snack:

The Healing Days

Days 1 and 2 of the plan are *healing* days. You treat your pouch like a newborn with gentle liquids and soups. Pouch inflammation is reduced and processed carbohydrate cravings subside. Mental focus is on listening to and respecting your body. Your menu on Days 1 and 2 mimics the early days and weeks following bariatric surgery. A diet of simple liquids, including protein drinks, clear broth, creamy soups, and hearty soups takes the guess work out of meal planning so you can focus on making *well* and making *right* your WLS tool.

> *Liquids are defined to include clear broth and creamy soups, protein fortified beverages, and hearty soups made of vegetables, legumes, and some animal protein and dairy.*

All meals on Days 1 and 2 are liquids as defined here. In the 5 Day Pouch Test liquids are defined to include clear broth and creamy soups, protein fortified beverages (protein shakes), and hearty soups made of vegetables, legumes with some animal protein and dairy. See the recipe section for delicious and healthy recipes to enjoy on Days 1 and 2. Many people find that including both protein fortified meal replacement shakes and the hearty soups in their diet on Days 1 and 2 improves their overall experience with the 5DPT. The purpose of all liquids is to disrupt snacking, grazing, or processed carbohydrate eating habits. In addition, the liquids will work to soothe and cleanse your system and prepare you for the following three days. Days 1 and 2 are all about pampering your pouch and healing your pouch from inflammation caused by poor dietary habits.

 Do not restrict food or caloric intake on the 5DPT

You can have as many liquid meals as needed in response to hunger or cravings. Some people are inclined to restrict food intake during the 5 Day Pouch Test: this is *not* encouraged because it leads to increased hunger cravings and frustration. *Do not restrict food intake: less is not better.* Pay close attention to the signals your body gives and when you are hungry eat something from the approved menu for the day. Soups are measured in 1-

cup servings and protein drinks are measured as the recipe or package directs. Stick with these portion sizes and eat what you can in 15 minutes. After 15 minutes discard what is uneaten and take pause to experience your pouch noting feelings of fullness and satiation. Wait at least one full hour before your next serving of liquid meal. Use this time to be mindful of your body; to get in touch with your pouch. Learning to feel the pouch and listening for authentic biological hunger signals is essential to your successful weight management. If you are truly hungry after waiting one hour, then have another serving of one of the approved meals. Again, take only 15 minutes to eat and continue to be alert to the signals your body sends.

Time all meals: 15 minutes

Many bariatric centers recommend patients take 30 minutes to eat meals. Some even instruct patients to use a stopwatch and time three minutes between bites of food. The reason is to slow down the eating habits of the recovering morbidly obese person. As the patient recovers from surgery and becomes more comfortable eating they tend to eat more volume and often continue to eat over the 30 minutes allowed for a meal, even though satiation has already been achieved. Eventually the caloric intake at meals increases in spite of the stomach pouch restrictions. This is particularly true for patients who introduce beverages back into their meal disregarding the liquid restrictions.

The point is not to see how close you can come to nausea. Learn to eat until satisfied, then stop eating and avoid getting sick.

During the pouch test a person is following the liquid restrictions and eating a high protein diet. By limiting meal time to 15 minutes one will enjoy the satisfying feeling that is the desired result of a gastric pouch. The following is from the Gastric Bypass Instructions from Alvarado Hospital:

"When you feel satisfied you are finished. Don't get trapped in the belief that you have to eat everything on your plate, or that you can't possibly get by with that small a meal. Your meals will be small, and they are supposed to be small. If you feel full and satisfied and you try to eat any more, you will begin to feel nauseated; and you may throw up. The point is not to see how close you can come to nausea. Learn to eat until satisfied and to avoid getting sick." (Wittgrove, 1999)

Protein Fortified Beverages: Protein shakes, protein drinks, protein breakfast drinks are all protein fortified beverages. Look for ready-to-drink (RTD) beverages that have at least 15 grams of protein and fewer than 5 grams of carbohydrate per serving. Protein powder drinks are acceptable as well, providing they meet the same criterion of 15 grams protein and fewer than 5 grams carbohydrate. Homemade protein smoothies are a favorable addition to the 5DPT menu. They can be created with or without protein powder using low-fat cottage cheese, yogurt and fruit or berries. See the recipe section. Each of us has a unique taste preference when it comes to protein beverages. You are responsible for finding the protein beverage you like and using it as part of your long-term weight management diet.

Clear broth or creamy soups: Clear broth and creamy soups are a favorite comfort food for many of us. Canned commercial chicken broth, beef broth, and vegetable broth are enjoyable meals on Days 1 and 2. Look for ready-to-eat broth that is low-sodium or reduced sodium and enjoy 1-cup servings. Do not drink any liquids for 30 minutes before or after having a warm cup of broth. Again, we want the pouch to absorb the nutrients from the food and we want to feel full as long as possible. Even though clear broth is a liquid of similar viscosity to water it contains nutrients and energy from which the body benefits.

You may find it beneficial to add a soup flavored or unflavored protein powder to your serving of soup or broth. Please note the instructions on your protein powder: most recommend using warm water of less than 130ºF degrees or the texture will be affected.

Swanson ready-to-eat 50% Less Sodium Beef Broth® is a good example of readily available commercial clear soup appropriate for the 5DPT. A 1-cup serving provides 15 calories, 3 grams protein, 1 grams carbohydrate, no fat and 400mg sodium. When shopping for a commercial soup, look for nutritional data that is comparable to this example. There are many good regional soups available at specialty food stores and larger supermarkets. Do some exploring and find something you can enjoy knowing you are feeding your body well.

A quality protein powder will add as many as 21 grams of protein to your 1-cup serving of soup. *Tip:* When you find a protein powder you like try including it in your meals as often as possible. Good quality protein supplementation is a terrific tool in our ongoing weight management strategy.

Creamy soups are a comfort food favorite for Days 1 and 2. Many creamy soups include dairy products such as milk, cream, sour cream, or half-and-half. For purposes of the 5DPT full-fat dairy should be used as called for in the Day 1 and 2 recipes because it improves satiation longer than no-fat or reduced fat food. *Note: After the 5DPT feel free to modify the soups with reduced or low-fat dairy as you find appropriate with your ongoing weight management. The soups are very good and always a welcome inclusion in a healthy Day 6 and beyond diet.* People with lactose intolerance[4] should avoid including creamy soups in their 5DPT and their regular diet. Select the hearty soups or clear broths instead.

Campbell's Healthy Request® Cream of Mushroom Soup is a good commercial soup that works well on the 5DPT. A 1-cup serving of soup prepared with 2% milk provides 130 calories, 6 grams protein, 5 grams fat (1 gram saturated), 10 grams carbohydrate, and 410mg sodium. For on-the-go meals try Campbell's Soup at Hand® 25% Less Sodium Classic Tomato Soup. Heated quickly in the microwave and served in the same container this convenient soup provides 140 calories, 3g protein, 0g fat, 33g carbohydrate and 480mg sodium. Use these examples to find ready-to-eat creamy soups you will enjoy including in your 5DPT and beyond.

The Dietary Guidelines for Americans created by the U.S. Department of Health and Human Services and the U.S. Department of Agriculture sets the recommended daily intake of sodium at 2300mg. Excess sodium is a contributory factor in the development of hypertension, which is a major risk factor for heart disease and stroke. (Institute of Medicine, 2010)

Hearty Soups: As I developed this plan I learned that more substantial soups made of animal protein, legumes, beans, and low-glycemic vegetables work well to alleviate the discomfort and stress of a liquid diet. These satisfying

---

[4] Lactose intolerance is a condition that results from inability to digest the milk sugar lactose; characterized by bloating, gas, abdominal discomfort, and diarrhea. Lactose intolerance may present in gastric surgery patients who did not have the condition prior to surgery. A lack of digestive enzyme is believed to be the cause. (Whitney & Rolfes, 2005)

soup recipes are made of foods low on the Glycemic Index (GI), a measure of how your blood glucose levels are affected by food. That means they will stick with you without causing a rapid rise and subsequent drop in blood glucose. These great comfort soups will help keep you feeling full longer, help you achieve and maintain a healthy weight, and provide you with more consistent energy throughout the day.

When including hearty soups as part of your 5DPT menu I encourage you to cook and enjoy the recipes provided. These recipes are specific to the plan and they work very well in our five day dietary progression. An added bonus: the soup recipes offered are less expensive per serving than prepared soups or protein drinks and they are family friendly making the 5 Day Pouch Test practical to incorporate into our busy schedules. Check out the recipe section for delicious soups and smoothies and make them a part of your LivingAfterWLS way of life.

Soups vs. Sliders: It is easy to confuse soup with slider foods since both are liquids that flow more rapidly through the stoma than solid protein. The thing to remember is the soup recipes provided are nutrient dense. Slider foods such as crackers or pretzels washed down with liquids have no nutritional value nor are they satiating. In addition, when we enjoy soup and observe the liquid restrictions our body benefits from the vitamins and nutrients in the meal while we enjoy a comforting feeling of satiation.

There are times when we will need to eat restaurant food during the 5 Day Pouch Test and on Day 6 and beyond. A carefully selected soup can be a favorable choice on the menu. Review these restaurant choices and look at their nutritional score. You can also find many restaurant menus online and they often contain nutritional values. Use these examples as guidelines and you will be ready to identify a comparable dish when eating a meal in a restaurant or fast food establishment.

On the menu look for:
1-cup soup servings with 8-21 grams protein; low-glycemic vegetables, beans and legumes that provide nutrient rich complex carbohydrates and dietary fiber; avoid all trans-fat; Sodium should be 1,000mg or lower. Soups made with fresh seasonal vegetables are always a good choice.

Panera Bread Low-Fat Vegetarian Black Bean Soup: A 1-cup serving provides 150 calories and 8 grams protein. That is a little low for protein requirements per meal but the soup also provides 6 grams of fiber while being low in fat and virtually trans-fat free. The carbs, measuring 28 grams per serving, seem high at first glance. But black beans are low-glycemic (GI Value 30) complex carbohydrates. Black beans are an ideal food for fighting carb cravings. They are rich in folate, manganese, thiamin (B vitamins) and potassium

Wendy's Cup of Chili: A small serving of Wendy's Chili (about 1 cup) provides 190 calories with 14 grams protein, 5 grams fiber, 19 grams carbohydrate (again - low GI), and is low in fat. The sodium comes in high at 830mg in this serving size. That is 36% of the recommended sodium intake of 2,300mg/day. Enjoy this tasty cup of chili in moderation and seek lower sodium food choices for other meals consumed that day.

Boston Market Chicken Noodle Soup: A 6-ounce serving provides 170 calories with 13 grams protein and 17 grams carbohydrate. Like most commercially prepared soups the sodium is high at 930mg per serving, 38% of your daily value. This is a broth based soup so it is very important to remember your liquid restrictions and avoid drinking fluids for 30 minutes before and 30 minutes after eating. This will help your pouch stay full longer and give your body a better opportunity to absorb the nutrients. One benefit of eating soups when dining out is that your mouth stays moist making conversation more pleasant without the inclusion of additional liquids during the meal.

Carbohydrate withdrawal and nausea

Carbohydrate withdrawal: When any heavily consumed food is withdrawn from the diet the body is likely to experience symptoms of withdrawal that may include headache, dizziness, cramping, and nausea. This is not unique to our WLS body; this is a simple fact of biology. On the 5DPT when processed carbs are withdrawn many people report symptoms of "carbohydrate withdrawal." Do not suffer through this. If you notice symptoms of carbohydrate withdrawal eat a small piece of melon, some berries, an apple or an orange. Any low-glycemic fruit or vegetable will reduce the symptoms of carbohydrate withdrawal.

You may also try a serving of Emergen-C® energy booster fizzy drink mix, which is known to reduce the symptoms and discomfort of carbohydrate withdrawal. In addition, Emergen-C® provides B vitamins for energy and C vitamins for immunity along with many other vitamins and minerals. You can count a serving of Emergen-C® as part of your daily intake of water. Do not be put off by the 5 or 6 grams carbohydrate per serving: these are beneficial nutrient dense big-bang-for-your-buck carbs. Enjoy!

For nausea, try sipping freshly brewed warm green tea or ginger herbal tea. You can add fresh ginger juice to further ease the symptoms of stomach distress and nausea. If you made the Fennel & Celery Soup (page 36) for a grumpy pouch and have some left then enjoy a 1-cup serving of this soup. It is a known remedy to digestive discomfort and distress resulting from dietary change.

Understanding the Glycemic Index (GI)

The Glycemic Index (GI) was originally developed as a research tool for people with diabetes. Carbohydrates are assigned a GI value based on how they affect blood glucose levels. Carbohydrates that break down quickly raise blood sugar levels quickly: these foods are considered high on the Glycemic Index. Our first choice when eating carbohydrates should be those with a low GI value. They take longer to digest and have less impact on our blood glucose levels. Low GI value carbohydrates keep us on an even keel. We are well served to include low GI carbohydrates in our diet after weight loss surgery. Fruits and vegetables with a low GI rating provide a variety of vitamins and minerals along with dietary fiber and flavor. On the 5DPT when one experiences discomfort from carbohydrate withdrawal eating a small serving of low GI fruit of vegetable often brings relief. This is a short list of fruits and vegetables to avoid and fruits and vegetables to include in your 5DPT and beyond:

Enjoy low-glycemic fresh fruit: apple, avocado, banana, blueberries, cantaloupe, grapefruit, kiwi fruit, lemon, lime, mango, orange, peach, pear, plum, raspberries, and strawberries.

Avoid these high glycemic fruits: fresh apricots, cherries, papaya, pineapple, rhubarb, and watermelon.

Enjoy low-glycemic dried fruit: apple, apricots, dates, and prunes.

Enjoy low-glycemic fresh vegetables: alfalfa sprouts, artichokes, arugula, asparagus, bean sprouts, bok choy, broccoli, Brussels sprouts, cabbage, carrots, cauliflower, celery, chili peppers, chives, corn, cucumber, eggplant, endive, fennel, garlic, ginger, green beans, herbs, leeks, lettuce, mushrooms, okra, peppers, radishes, scallions, shallots, snow pea sprouts, spinach, squash, Swiss chard, tomato, turnip, watercress, and zucchini.

Avoid these high glycemic vegetables: beets, fava beans, parsnips, peas, potatoes, sweet potatoes, and yams.

Leading online resource: Glycemic Index

GlycemicIndex.com: Official website for the glycemic index and international GI database which is based in the Human Nutrition Unit, School of Molecular Biosciences, University of Sydney. The website is updated and maintained by the University's GI Group which includes research scientists and dietitians working in the area of glycemic index, health and nutrition including research into diet and weight loss, diabetes, cardiovascular disease and PCOS. http://www.glycemicindex.com/

The 5DPT is a carefully structured plan that continues to help countless thousands around the world return to their WLS basics. Here are a few reasons it works so effectively:

First: By retracing the early dietary stages that we followed post-surgery we enter a mental mindset of confidence and excitement. We capture the feelings we enjoyed in the early days and weeks following surgery when, for the first time in our dieting life, we were succeeding with a plan. Often frustrated post-WLS patients are told by their surgeons or nutritionists, *"You just need to get back to basics."* Indeed. We *know* we need to get back to basics, we just do not know how. Having a plan brings imminent success. Knowing the plan has worked for so many others since it was introduced in 2007 boosts our confidence that we can do this; this will work! The 5 Day Pouch Test gives us a starting point and a detailed method to get back to basics.

Inspired: "I can't explain how great it is to be in control again. I am walking more upright. I have found the spark that I had back when I first had my surgery. Thank You!" (Stephanie, 2009)

Second: A high protein diet increases the metabolism because protein requires the greatest amount of energy to burn. Nutritionists say protein has a high thermic effect: it requires more calories to digest than the calories it contains. Conversely, after digesting carbohydrate and fat nutrients extra calories from the food are leftover and available to be stored as adipose, the body's fat tissue, for future energy needs. This is the reason that the first rule of post-weight loss surgery is **Protein First**. That means protein must account for two-thirds of our dietary intake for all meals. Follow this rule and keep your metabolism in high thermic burn for effective weight management. Think of your adipose as the energy you saved for a rainy day. When your body needs more energy than provided on a high protein diet it withdraws from your rainy day fund to burn some of that stored body fat tissue: weight is lost.

Third: The elimination of processed carbohydrates and nutritionally void snack foods from the diet stabilizes the blood glucose level (blood sugar level). When we digest carbohydrates they are converted to glucose. The glucose goes to the liver and from there is released to our circulatory system:

the bloodstream. Processed carbs, also called slider foods, cause our blood glucose level to rise. When the glucose level returns to normal the body receives a message that more carbohydrates are needed and a craving or hunger signal is sent to the brain. So we reach for quick fix processed carbohydrates and the cycle continues. Maintaining a low blood glucose level with a high protein diet and carefully selected low glycemic fruits and vegetables will break this carb-cycle and improve our overall well-being.

Days 1 & 2 Key Learning Points

- Heal your pouch with soothing comforting liquids that are nutrient dense and low glycemic.
- Time your meals: 15 minutes per meal.
- Make informed dietary choices when eating at home, commercially prepared food or eating out.
- Do not suffer through carbohydrate withdrawal. Low glycemic fruits and vegetables reduce discomfort. Also try herbal tea or Emergen-C®.
- Revisit the empowerment you enjoyed after surgery: you are a powerful and capable person and you are getting back on track!

5 Day Pouch Test Journal: Days 1 & 2

Reclaim the power of your pouch and renew your commitment to healthy weight management with weight loss surgery. Use this tool daily so you can return to it often as a record of what you have learned, what you have achieved, and where you can go beyond the 5DPT. *(see next page)* See the appendix for a blank 5-page 5DPT Journal. If you prefer a full 8x11-inch worksheet visit 5DayPouchTest.com and click "Tools" for a free download.

Day 1 Journal: Liquids

The first two days are all liquids as defined in this plan. Monitor all food and beverage intake. Do your best! Take your vitamins, supplements, and prescription medications as directed by your health care provider. Exercise as your health and energy level allows. Continue building your storm of enthusiasm! You are powerful and you can do this!

Records:	Nutritional Intake – All food and Beverages				
Day/Date: *Weight:*	*Item*	*Pro(g)*	*Fat(g)*	*Carbs(g)*	*Calories*
Water Goal: 0 0 0 0 0 0 0 0 0 0 *Mark 1 bubble for each 8-ounce serving water.*					
Vitamins/Supplements:					
Exercise & Fitness:					
Goals/ *Totals:*					
Summary:					

Download 8.5x11" journal at 5DayPouchTest.com – Click Tools
See appendix for journal Days 1-5 for your use.

Day 2 Journal: Liquids

Day 2: You are on your way! Continue to monitor all food and beverage intake. Do your best! Take your vitamins, supplements, and prescription medications as directed by your health care provider. Exercise as your health and energy level allows. Continue building your storm of enthusiasm! You are powerful and you can do this!

Records:	Nutritional Intake – All food and Beverages				
Day/Date: Weight:	Item	Pro(g)	Fat(g)	Carbs(g)	Calories
Water Goal: 0 0 0 0 0 0 0 0 0 0 Mark 1 bubble for each 8-ounce serving water.					
Vitamins/Supplements:					
Exercise & Fitness:					
Goals/ Totals:					

Summary:

These are a few of the most Frequently Asked Questions about Days 1 and 2 of the 5 Day Pouch Test. Use this as a quick reference but always return to the text of the full plan for complete instruction.

Can I repeat the liquid days instead of going to Day 3?

You can repeat the liquid eating plan of the 5DPT Days 1 and 2, but as soon as you do that you are doing a liquid diet; *you are not doing the 5 Day Pouch Test.* The intent of the 5DPT is to quickly progress through the post-op dietary stages and get us back to the basics of following our weight loss surgery high protein, low carbohydrate diet. People are sometimes tempted to repeat the liquid days because they have recorded a pleasing weight loss on Days 1 and 2. Keep in mind this weight loss is primarily water loss. In order to keep losing weight one needs to follow a high protein diet that elevates the metabolism into high thermic burn: *this is when true weight is lost.*

We do not have to manage our plate with an all or nothing strategy: this has never worked for keeping our obesity under control. We must find the happy place between perfection and imperfection.

Please follow the 5DPT as it is written: it was developed to help you achieve the best results with your weight loss surgery. *We tested it numerous times so you don't have to.*

I messed up on Day 1: Should I start over to get it perfect?

I have never done the 5DPT perfectly and I do not know anyone who has. Rather than make the five days about perfection make this time about learning. Little mistakes will not stop the world from turning. So forge ahead doing your very best and forgive little mistakes. Learn from each day, review the key learning points and make notes on your 5 Day Pouch Test Journal. Emerge on Day 6 knowing more about yourself and how to work your tool. *You can do this!* One of the biggest dietary mistakes we make is thinking we must be totally perfect or totally imperfect. *We do not have to manage our plate with an all or nothing strategy: this has never worked for keeping our obesity under control.* Start thinking about doing your best in the moment and on the day and celebrate the little moments. Our LivingAfterWLS motto embraces this: *"Stop for a moment. Look where you are: You Have Arrived."*

Now is everything. Never forget that perfection is not the goal in anything: doing our best on the day and in the moment is *always* the goal.

Whatever else you have on your mind,
Wherever else you think you are going,
Stop for a moment.
Look where you are.
You Have Arrived!

How can soups with beans and meat work for a liquid diet?

The 5 Day Pouch Test calls for two days of protein rich liquids. Normally we think of ready-to-drink protein beverages or homemade concoctions using fruit, yogurt and protein powders as dietary liquids. This is quite typical of the early post-op diet prescribed by many surgical weight loss centers. The 5DPT begins with two days of protein liquids in order to baby the pouch, much as we did immediately post-op. In addition, the liquids are useful in breaking a processed carbohydrate snacking habit or slider food addiction. *(Review "Understanding the Liquid Options" earlier in this chapter.)*

Are dairy products okay to use on the 5DPT?

If you can tolerate milk and dairy products include them in your 5DPT and beyond. See the recipe section. Many WLS patients become lactose intolerant so that is why there is always a caution about using milk products. For those who can tolerate dairy, when used in moderation, it can be a healthy part of your diet.

Are yogurts or cottage cheese allowed on Days 1 & 2?

No, cottage cheese and yogurt should not be used as stand-alone menu choices on Days 1 and 2. However, they may be used as ingredients in protein smoothies. You can introduce yogurt and cottage cheese to your diet on Day 3: Soft Protein.

What is wrong with carbonated-caffeinated beverages?

There are a few reasons carbonated-caffeinated beverages are discouraged. First, they have no nutritional value and beverages that contain caffeine can cause dehydration. There is also the theory that for the body to absorb the carbonation bubbles oxygen is released from the blood stream to hook-up with the oxide molecules to be eliminated through the kidneys and urine. When oxygen levels in the blood go down so does our energy level and our metabolism slows. Finally, recent studies suggest the bubbles stretch the pouch outlet causing permanent dilation of the stoma which leads to regaining weight. (Barham K. Abu Dayyeh, 2011) More importantly, carbonated caffeine-containing beverages are void of nutritional value so why put them in our body?

Why is Emergen-C® fizzy drink allowed?

Most bariatric centers discourage patients from having bubbly carbonated beverages after surgery. The carbonation may cause discomfort in the pouch, may cause the pouch to expand temporarily and may cause temporary or lasting injury to the stoma. In addition, consumption of carbonated beverages generally means empty calories that are eaten with non-nutritional snack foods (think of the ubiquitous movie snack of a soda and popcorn). A fizzy vitamin drink mix is bubbly due to the effervescent reaction when the minerals react with the liquid. The fizz is not the result of pressurized carbon dioxide gas being forced into a liquid as is carbonation. Emergen-C® is an approved vitamin and mineral dietary supplement by most bariatric nutritionists. Some patients prefer to allow the effervescent bubbles to

Effervescent is not carbonation: effervescent is the fizzy bubbly result of minerals reacting with a liquid.

dissipate before drinking the vitamin mix. The rapid absorption of vitamins and minerals dissolved in water is an effective means for patients with malabsorption to take vitamin supplements.

Why do I need to reduce my coffee or caffeine intake?

Studies and opinions regarding caffeine change frequently in the study of health and nutrition. It has long been believed that caffeine is a diuretic or a substance that causes the body to lose fluid and disrupts the body's water balance, which is vital to our digestive, circulatory, and metabolic systems. This can slow weight loss, lead to thirst, fatigue, and weakness. Some believe there is no nutritional value to caffeine and it can be addictive. Those wishing to eliminate or reduce their caffeine intake should do so gradually. Going cold turkey may cause headaches, irritability, nausea, and other symptoms. Doctors say that if you want to reduce the amount of caffeine you consume, slow down gradually to avoid these withdrawal symptoms. Please stay current with your reading regarding caffeine and nutrition and always seek the advice of your health care professional regarding your individual nutritional needs.

Does that mean drinking coffee will defeat the 5DPT?

Coffee will not defeat the 5 Day Pouch Test. But if you are interested in reducing your coffee and/or caffeine intake now is a good time to gradually cut back.

Can I have sugar free gum or candy on the 5DPT?

Refer to your original post-surgery dietary instructions to see if sugar free gum and candy are recommended for patients with your procedure. Sugar free products are typically made with sugar alcohols that contribute to digestive distress including gas, bloating, and diarrhea. Many bariatric nutritionists discourage patients from including sugar free sweets in the post-WLS diet. Please follow the recommendations of your bariatric team.

My spouse/partner/friend wants to do the 5DPT with me and they have not had the surgery.
Is it okay if they do it with me?

It is great to have a supportive spouse or friend and a normal tummy (non-WLS individual) doing the 5DPT will not be harmed. However, they do not have the benefit of pouch restriction and may experience hunger with the portion restrictions. Have them follow the FDA guidelines for serving size and avoid the higher fat soups that could be over-consumed. A note, many non-surgical testers of the 5DPT report that following the liquid restrictions results in less food consumption. Never diminish the value of having a teammate in the 5DPT; welcome all willing participants and embrace their encouragement. We are all in this together.

What does 'broken my pouch' mean?

In the early weeks and months following gastric surgery there is a distinct feeling of tightness in the small stomach pouch created by the surgery. Small meals of dense protein and void of starch quickly bring a full feeling to a new post-op patient. This tightness triggers satiation for the patient: a strong signal of fullness. Weight loss results because of the decreased caloric consumption affected by the small gastric pouch.

As patients get further out from surgery there is a tendency to experiment with the pouch, perhaps including liquids with meals or eating foods that exit the pouch quickly, commonly called slider foods. In the worst case slider foods are consumed with liquid; an example is graham crackers and coffee. In this case the coffee and graham crackers create slurry in the pouch and slide right through the outlet to the intestine, thus never filling the pouch. Caught quite unaware patients ask, *"Is my pouch broken?"* They report their pouch does not feel the same tightness as it did early post-op when the pouch was new and they were compliant with the prescribed way of eating. When patients do the 5 Day Pouch Test they are surprised to feel the pouch again simply by returning to the way of eating that worked in the first place after surgery.

Chapter 5: Day 3 - Soft Protein

Feeling the tightness again.

As on Days 1 and 2, for the next three days you get to eat as much as you want as often as you want. But there is a catch: you must follow the plan. Again there are specific menu choices for Day 3. Today we introduce soft protein served in carefully measured portions. After two days of 5DPT liquids the introduction of soft protein is a welcome dietary change. It is likely on Day 3 you will start to feel that "newbie" tightness in your pouch. In addition, your hunger or carb cravings are likely to be diminished. Continue to observe the liquid restrictions and take your meals only on a "dry" pouch. Your dry pouch will hold soft protein longer prolonging feelings of satiety.

Protein Recommendations Day 3: canned fish (tuna or salmon) mixed with lemon and seasoned with salt and pepper, eggs cooked as desired seasoned with salt pepper and/or salsa, fresh soft fish (tilapia, sole, orange roughy), baked or grilled, and lightly seasoned. Yogurt and cottage cheese are allowed in ½-cup servings, and 1-ounce cheese servings, such as string cheese, are an acceptable between-meal snack provided liquid restrictions are followed. Vegetarian animal protein replacement products such as tofu or vegetable and legume patties are acceptable on Day 3.

Measure your portion (1-cup volume or 4 to 6-ounces weight) and eat only until you feel full, not stuffed. If you need to add a moist condiment (mayonnaise, mustard, relish, salsa and the like) to the canned fish I understand, but keep it to a measured serving as indicated on the product label. A universal favorite for Day 3 is the Parmesan Tuna Patties from the recipe section: make it and enjoy! I bet you find this recipe on your menu far beyond the 5DPT. Substitute canned chicken or turkey if you have an aversion to canned fish.

As a rule on Day 3 fish is the preferred menu option because it is softer and moister than canned poultry. In addition, fish canned in water is considered low fat, a direction we are heading during the 5DPT. However, the chicken and poultry will take on a softer texture when prepared according to the recipes provided and it will work in much the same way as canned fish. And never underestimate the egg dishes and breakfast bakes for any meal on Day

3. These are tasty, economical, and family friendly recipes that are delicious any time and sure to become favorites on Day 6 and beyond. As you advance to Days 4 and 5 you may enjoy any leftovers from your Day 3 recipes. Please take a look at the recipe section.

The 5DPT is a program of advancing our diet following the same dietary progression we were instructed to follow immediately after surgery. That means you can always advance foods from the early stages (Days 1 and 2 for example) to the later stages (Days 3, 4, and 5). If a food was allowed for Days 1 and 2 you can enjoy the same food as part of your menu during the next three days and beyond. For best results meals should be from the menu plan on the day. Snack options may come from the earlier days of the 5DPT.

Surrender to the change

Erase this sentence from your vocabulary: *"I don't deal well with change."* When we signed on to have weight loss surgery we authorized the highest level of change any dieter will ever submit to: surgical intervention.

In the course of his studies on evolution Charles Darwin discovered that in sea turtles it is not the strongest of the species that survive, nor is it the most intelligent of the species that survive. The survivors are those most responsive to change. As weight loss surgery patients we have affected a major change on our bodies, our species. I consider that we caused a voluntary acceleration of evolution and because of this we must embrace and accept change with great enthusiasm: we cannot go back. We have forsaken the right to say, *"I don't deal well with change."*

We don't have to be the strongest or most intelligent: we simply have to move forward accepting this change and find what works.

Following Darwin's observation we understand that we don't have to be the strongest or most intelligent to survive and thrive: we simply have to move forward accepting this change and find what works.

Our surgeons have skillfully changed us physically: medical evolution if you will. But the more difficult change comes from within: within our mind; our heart; and yes, our spiritual being. When we embrace inner change our physical being will follow.

As part of embracing change I ask you to be kind to yourself.

Be kind to yourself.

This is a fundamental tenet of the 5 Day Pouch Test and LivingAfterWLS. Often people recovering from morbid obesity *(myself included)* put us last on the priority list. Anything else feels selfish and we are giving people, right? Yet diminishing our wellness and needs prevents us from being our best. We cannot give fully of ourselves until we are healthy inside and out.

By Day 3 of the 5DPT you are well on your way to returning to your post-surgery way of life, the life that was a complete and dramatic change from anything you experienced before surgery. Surrender to the change, the rules, and the requirements. You will find freedom in this surrender and you will be in control of pursuing the healthy life you only hoped for before undergoing surgery.

Focus: Practice mental presence

Practice mental presence during the 5 Day Pouch Test: be mindful of what you eat; how you move your body; and how your energy levels rise and fall. Be completely aware of yourself and identify the things that are working and helping you feel refreshed and alive. Use the 5 Day Pouch Test journal to record your experience and focus on learning about yourself. Awareness is not selfish; it is part of the process of understanding so that we may improve our health and wellness. Carry this focus forward to Day 6 and continue to treat your body in a kind and healthy manner and avoid stepping back into the self-loathing and unhealthy behavior that brought you here.

Awareness is not selfish; it is part of the process of understanding so that we may improve our health and wellness.

Rethink the way we eat

Now that you have made it through the difficult liquid days you can start to think about ways to use the things you are learning on the 5DPT on Day 6 and beyond. A popular Day 3 recipe is the Cranberry Turkey Roll-Ups (see recipe section) which takes three ingredients to build a terrific on-the-go meal that is satisfying, affordable, and simply delicious. This recipe is offered not because it is a magic formula for weight loss. It is offered because it is delicious and it meets our dietary needs as WLS-patients who are living in the real world. When we learn to work our tool in the real world we are winning the battle. Use the 5DPT as your vehicle to LivingAfterWLS in the real world.

Low-Sodium Meat & Cheese: The deli counter is a great source of meat and cheese that support our high protein diet. You can buy only the amount you need freshly sliced or select from brand name prepackaged sliced meats. Deli meat and cheese are great for on-the-go meals and make sense for snacking as well. Here are a few ideas that work for me:

Deli Roll-ups: Take one or two slices of deli meat (depending on thickness), spread with whipped cream cheese, top with a half-slice of cheese and roll-up; secure with a toothpick. Enjoy at once or wrap tightly in plastic wrap and refrigerate for later. Make several at a time assembly line fashion to be ready to grab on the way out the door.

Consider these nutritionals for one average serving of our not so average deli roll-ups: Take 4 slices (2-ounces) Hormel Natural Choice Oven Roasted Deli Turkey, 2 Tablespoons Philadelphia whipped cream cheese and 1 (1-ounce) slice (divided) provolone cheese: Make 2 roll-ups. Each two roll-up serving provides 220 calories; 18 grams protein; 15 grams fat; 4 grams carbohydrate; 655mg sodium (28% RDI). Enjoy with a pickle on the side and laugh in the face of a bread-happy deli sandwich: you are the envy of all at your picnic table. Enjoy lunch and thrive all afternoon fully alert without the burden of a carb-heavy meal taking you down. That is *living*!

Clever add-ins: Jam or jelly, pickle-relish, chopped veggies stirred into the whipped cream cheese, olives, pickles, roasted red peppers. Follow your taste cravings and explore an exciting new world of roll-ups the WLS high protein way.

Eating out on Day 3

In spite of our best laid plans to dedicate five days to our health and lifestyle management with weight loss surgery the simple fact is we may need to eat out along the way. Restaurants are yielding to public pressure and offering more healthy selections that are trans-fat free, lower in fat, lighter on the starch and non-nutritional carbs. Now, more than ever before, we have access to nutritional information for menu choices at many national chain restaurants. We have the advantage of learning what is offered thus making it easier to select a healthy meal when ordering.

Of course, it is best to avoid eating out during these five days but just in case you must, planning ahead to make informed choices serves our best interest.

During the 5DPT please avoid eating more than one restaurant meal a day and try not to have more than three restaurant meals during the 5 day plan. *This advice isn't disciplinary:* this is simply good wisdom for making the most of your effort so that you will enjoy success and empowerment. For our purposes on Day 3 of the 5DPT here are some selections that may be worked into our meal plan for the day.

Long John Silvers: Baked Cod. 1 piece provides 120 calories; 22 grams protein; 5 grams fat; 1 gram carbohydrate, 240 mg sodium.

Bob Evans Restaurants: Potato Crusted Flounder. 1 serving provides 254 calories; 17 grams protein; 17 grams fat; 8 grams carbohydrate; 552mg sodium.

Bob Evans Restaurants: Farmer's Market Omelet with Egg Lites. Enjoy only what you can eat of this generous serving. A full serving provides 544 calories; 38 grams protein; 35 grams fat; 13 grams carbohydrate; 1883mg sodium.

Romano's Macaroni Grill. Parmesan Crusted Sole – Lunch Serving. Enjoy only what you can eat of this generous serving. Avoid eating any other high sodium food on the day you enjoy this. A full serving provides 1800 calories; 47 grams protein; 52 grams fat; 106 grams carbohydrate; 3220mg sodium.

Blimpie Subs and Salads: Tuna Salad (Regular). 1 serving provides 272 calories; 18 grams protein; 6 grams fat; 7 grams carbohydrate; 517mg sodium.

This is a small sample of choices available when eating out. When you know where you will be eating in advance visit the website and make your menu selection, write it down or type it into your phone. At the restaurant decline the menu –*those photos are so tempting*—and place your order as you pre-planned it. Try this just once and you will revel in how powerful you feel. Then enjoy your meal without feeling disappointed in yourself; you triumphed!

- Surrender to change. This is what it takes to survive. Weight loss surgery affects a profound change on the body. Now is your chance to let your mind catch-up and embrace that change.
- Practice mental presence.
- Rethinking the way we eat. When we learn to work our tool in the real world we are winning the battle. Use the 5DPT as your vehicle to LivingAfterWLS in the real world!
- In this age of instant information access, we have the advantage of looking online at restaurant menus before ever going out to eat. A little reconnaissance work gives us the power to make informed choices when ordering our meal. There is a triumphant feeling that comes with living in the real world and making our WLS work at the same time.

Day 3 Journal: Soft Protein

Day 3 introduces soft protein including eggs, fish, and seafood. Monitor all food and beverage intake. Your momentum is unstoppable. Take your vitamins, supplements, and prescription medications as directed by your health care provider. Exercise as your health and energy level allows. Continue building your storm of enthusiasm! You can do this!

Records:	Nutritional Intake – All food and Beverages				
Day/Date: Weight:	Item	Pro(g)	Fat(g)	Carbs(g)	Calories
Water Goal: 0 0 0 0 0 0 0 0 0 0 Mark 1 bubble for each 8-ounce serving water.					
Vitamins/Supplements:					
Exercise & Fitness:					
Goals/ Totals:					
Summary:					

Download 8.5x11" journal at 5DayPouchTest.com – Click Tools
See appendix for journal Days 1-5 for your use.

These are a few of the most Frequently Asked Questions about Day 3 of the 5 Day Pouch Test. Many of these questions are addressed throughout the plan: use this as a quick reference but always return to the text of the full plan for complete instruction.

On Day 3 can I have refried beans?

You can have refried beans on Day 3. They are low- glycemic and protein dense. Be sure and measure your portion; no more than ½-cup. You get 8 grams of protein in ½-cup so try to include another protein source such as an egg for 7 more grams of protein. In fact, a great breakfast on Day 3 is the Mock Breakfast Burrito; take a look at the recipe section.

Always be cautious when eating cooked beans or legumes of any kind and measure your portion at no more than ½-cup. It seems the beans tend to expand once mastication occurs and digestion begins. Eating a larger portion of cooked beans or legumes may cause discomfort including gas, bloating, diarrhea, and/or vomiting.

Is Wendy's chili for lunch on Day 3 a good choice?

Wendy's chili is a popular and acceptable choice for Day 3 of the 5DPT. A small serving of Wendy's Chili (about 1 cup – see note above regarding beans and serving size) provides 190 calories with 14 grams protein, 5 grams fiber, 19 grams carbohydrate *(again - low GI)*, and is low in fat. The sodium comes in high at 830mg in the small serving size. That is 36% of the recommended sodium intake of 2,300mg/day. Enjoy this tasty cup of chili in moderation.

Can I have protein shakes on Days 3, 4 and 5?

You can include protein drinks on Days 3 to 5, but only as between meal snacks if you are hungry. It is best to stick with the menu foods, but on the other hand, if you are hungry or "*snacky*" go for the protein shake. It will raise your metabolism and satiate your hunger. A protein drink counts as a meal so follow the liquid restrictions. Let your body get the full benefit of this protein and vitamin fortified meal by not washing it down with liquids. Also, if you have scheduled a protein drink in your eating plan take your vitamin supplements with it for better digestion and absorption. When in doubt mindfully enjoy a protein drink first before eating any other snack food. *Remember this trick!* Even beyond the 5DPT a protein drink is always the best first choice for in between meals snack. A protein drink will serve your snacking needs well without derailing your best efforts for healthy weight management after WLS.

Ponder this: I'm not the number one fan of protein drinks but I include them in my diet for the nutritional benefit and the convenience. At times when I'm feeling hungry between meals and I give myself the choice between a protein shake or waiting it out I chose to wait. And I'm just fine. For times when you just cannot go without nourishment any longer do take a long pour of the protein shake and feed your body well avoiding a frantic reach into the snack bag.

More often than not our feelings of hunger are not an emergency and we can make it quite well to the next meal without a frantic reach into the snack bag or rapid pour of the protein shake.

When can I have a protein bar?

Protein bars can be included in your diet on Days 3, 4, and 5 of the 5 Day Pouch Test. Be mindful of the liquid restrictions and avoid consuming beverages as you enjoy your protein bar. Many protein bars are dry and cause thirst. We often turn to warm beverages, such as coffee or cocoa, to wash them down. This turns an otherwise healthy protein-smart choice into a slider food and missed opportunity for nutrient absorption. See "ponder this" in the FAQ above. Select protein bars that have at least 15 grams of protein and fewer than 6 grams of carbohydrate.

Help! I'm craving peanut butter!

Are you a person who craves peanut butter? Many people report strong cravings for peanut butter while doing the 5DPT. Peanut butter is one of those innocent things that can get us into trouble. Have you ever simply eaten peanut butter from the jar? No measuring or preparation, just a spoonful here or there? I am guilty! Those random tastes add lots of calories without the benefit of meal-time satiation. If you crave peanut butter, include it in a more mindful manner by making and enjoying my recipe for Mocha Peanut Butter Bites. See the recipe section.

Doing the 5DPT caused constipation. Is this normal?

A protein-dense diet naturally contains less dietary fiber than a high-carbohydrate diet. When the body metabolizes protein there is little waste to be eliminated, therefore feelings of constipation result. Here are suggestions to help relieve those feelings:

- 1/2 apple with skin for your mid-morning and mid-afternoon snack
- Increase your fluid intake
- Include a water-soluble fiber supplement in your daily diet
- Add a fish oil capsule to your diet
- Drink an herbal tea that contains senna leaf, hibiscus leaf, licorice root, and/or rhubarb root. Look for a specific laxative tea blend.
- Prepare one of the Feed the Carb Monster Soups for days 1 & 2 (each 1-cup serving contains 5 grams dietary fiber) and use this soup for a snack on Days 3, 4, and 5.
- Keep in mind that a high protein diet simply does not produce as much waste as a diet high in carbohydrates and fat. Your bathroom patterns are likely to change when following a high protein diet.
- Always address concerns about chronic constipation with your bariatric center or general medical care provider.

No Vegetables on the 5DPT? Why?

One of the most frequently asked questions from those doing the 5 Day Pouch Test is, "Why can't I have vegetables on the 5DPT?" This is understandable. Vegetables are a good source of vitamins, nutrients, flavor, and fiber. They play an important role in our healthy diet.

Vegetables are to be used only as ingredients in meal preparation, such as salsa on grilled fish or the Carb Monster Soups. By restricting vegetables and fruit (complex carbohydrates) during the five days your body is forced to go into high metabolic burn to digest the protein. This should result in weight loss. In addition, restricting complex carbohydrates and eliminating processed carbohydrates helps regulate your blood sugar (glucose) preventing cravings and energy swings.

Vegetables and low-glycemic fruit should be gradually introduced back to the diet on Day 6 and beyond. The focus must always remain on Protein First. A portion-controlled high-protein diet is how we lose weight after a surgical gastric procedure, and that is how we can maintain a healthy weight for the rest of our life.

Chapter 6: Day 4- Firm Proteins

Your new normal.

By Day 4 the carbohydrate cycle is broken and the liquid restrictions are becoming a habit. Most people report a genuine feeling of pouch-tightness, as they emerge ready to enjoy firm protein. Our Day 4 meals and eating habits are starting to feel like the new normal. And indeed, this is the way we need to eat in order to manage our weight after surgery. Our meals should be Protein First enjoyed with small portions of well-chosen vegetables and fruits. Remember the 2B/1B Rhythm: 2 Bites Protein, 1 Bite Complex Carbohydrate. Take time to chew every bite, resting the fork between bites, and enjoy the meal. Observe the liquid restrictions in order to achieve fullness and benefit from the nutrients in our food. Avoid slider foods and snacking on non-nutritional belly-filler foods. Welcome to Day 4: Today is your new normal.

Day 4 protein recommendations: ground meat (beef, turkey, lamb, game) cooked dry and lightly seasoned; shellfish, scallops, lobster, steamed and seasoned only with lemon; salmon, or halibut steaks, grilled and lightly seasoned. Vegetarian products including tofu and vegetable burgers are acceptable. Be sure to give the Salisbury Steak recipe a try and keep it in your menu rotation well beyond the 5 Day Pouch Test.

By now you should be experiencing that familiar tightness that will assure you that your pouch is working. Remember to drink plenty of water between meals. Take some time to appreciate the power of your pouch. Often we don't like that uncomfortable tightness in the pouch after eating just a few bites of firm protein without liquids. The tightness is reminiscent of a post-Thanksgiving feast that leads to a gluttony-induced nap. It is this tightness that makes the surgery work. And ironically, it is this tightness that leads us unaware back to slider foods, which do not cause discomfort: they sit better and we can prolong the enjoyment of eating.

On Day 4 and forever in your new normal the discomfort in your pouch is the signal to stop eating. This is the new normal. Concentrate today on how your pouch feels and put the fork down at the first sign of fullness. Stop short of the discomfort. This is how the weight loss surgery tool is meant to work. This is how you, the owner of the tool, can optimize the performance of the tool. I hope you are rediscovering your tool and enjoying relief and excitement knowing your pouch still works.

Breakfast Solutions Days 4 and 5

Traditional breakfast usually means whole grains, dairy and fruit or juice. The focus on a high protein breakfast presents a challenge to our traditional practices. The 5DPT is a good time to look outside of the cereal box for high protein choices. Protein first thing in the morning is a great way to raise our metabolic thermostat because it takes a lot of energy to metabolize protein. More importantly, a breakfast of 70% protein or more will stabilize our blood sugar and prevent hunger cravings. Here are some ideas:

Eggs, leftover tuna patties from Day 3, measured portions of cottage cheese or yogurt, peel-and-eat shrimp, ground beef, chicken, or turkey patties grilled or broiled, each provide ample protein to start the day. And of course, in a pinch, we can always count on protein drinks or meal replacement bars for the first meal of the day.

Understanding Hunger: Learning the signals

Hunger is not the only physiological signal managing our food intake. There are several factors that decide when it is time to eat and when it is time to stop eating. As recovering morbidly obese people it is important to understand the signals our body sends in order to lose weight and not become morbidly obese again. After all, ignoring these signals contributed to our obesity in the first place.

The following definitions are from Understanding Nutrition (Whitney & Rolfes, 2005), pages 252-256:

Hunger: the painful sensation caused by a lack of food that initiates food-seeking behavior.

Hypothalamus (high-po-THAL-ah-mus): a brain center that controls activities such as maintenance of water balance, regulation of body temperature, and control of appetite.

Appetite: the integrated response to the sight, smell, thought, or taste of food that initiates or delays eating.

Satiation (say-she-AY-shun): the feeling of satisfaction and fullness that occurs during a meal and halts eating. Satiation determines how much food is consumed during a meal.

Satiety (sah-TIE-eh-tee): the feeling of satisfaction that occurs after a meal and inhibits eating until the next meal. Satiety determines how much time passes between meals.

There are three types of influences that trigger hunger: physical, sensory and cognitive.

The most reliable influence is physical: an empty stomach, gastric contractions, and the absence of nutrients in the small intestine, gastrointestinal hormones and endorphins. Sensory influences such as the thought, sight, smell and taste of food will trigger hunger. And finally, perhaps the influence we know best, cognitive. That is the presence of others, special occasions, perception of hunger (head hunger), the time of day or the presence of food. In other words, external cues.

But as we all know, there are mental and external cues that can lead to hunger, appetite, and even satiety. According to Understanding Nutrition, "Eating can be triggered by signals other than hunger, even when the body does not need food. Some people experience food cravings when they are bored or anxious. In fact, they may eat in response to any kind of stress, negative or positive. These cognitive influences can easily lead to weight gain." (Whitney & Rolfes, 2005)

As we go forward with our post-surgical weight loss living it is important to pay attention to the feelings of satiation and satiety. The small stomach works well (when used correctly) to signal a feeling of satiation and indicate it is time to stop eating. This leads to satiety, which is like a pink sticky note that reminds us to not start eating again.

Develop a new awareness and listen to your body. Finally, just as hunger is not an emergency, it is also not a failure. If you feel hunger during the 5 Day Pouch Test carefully assess the signals to decide the state of urgency. After careful assessment if you are still hungry then eat something from the approved list of foods for the day. Associating hunger with feelings of failure often leads to destructive eating and inappropriate food choices. *Feeling hunger is not a moral problem*: it is simply a small part of a very complicated biological process.

- This is our new normal: the way we will eat to manage our health and weight with weight loss surgery. The Four Rules are now a way of life and a matter of habit.
- Look beyond the breakfast cereal box to feed your body at the beginning of the day.
- As recovering morbidly obese people it is important to understand the signals our body sends in order to lose weight and not become morbidly obese again. After all, ignoring these signals contributed to our obesity in the first place.
- **Feeling hunger is not a moral problem**: it is one small part of a very complicated biological process. The 5DPT is a powerful tool and a great step toward building a better relationship with food and your weight loss surgery.

Notes: My New Normal

Day 4 Journal: Firm Protein

Day 4 brings food back to the table. Remember to chew, chew, chew. Monitor all food and beverage intake. Do your best! Take your vitamins, supplements, and prescription medications as directed by your health care provider. Today you should feel more energy: add exercise and motion to your day. This is your new normal. You are powerful and you can do this!

Records:	Nutritional Intake – All food and Beverages				
Day/Date: Weight:	Item	Pro(g)	Fat(g)	Carbs(g)	Calories
Water Goal: 0 0 0 0 0 0 0 0 0 0 Mark 1 bubble for each 8-ounce serving water.					
Vitamins/Supplements:					
Exercise & Fitness:					
Goals/ Totals:					
Summary:					

Download 8.5x11" journal at 5DayPouchTest.com – Click Tools
See appendix for journal Days 1-5 for your use.

These are a few of the most Frequently Asked Questions about Day 4 of the 5 Day Pouch Test. Many of these questions are addressed throughout the plan: use this as a quick reference but always return to the text of the full plan for complete instruction.

I'm on Day 4 and only lost 2 pounds
What am I doing wrong?

First, please keep in mind the 5 Day Pouch Test is not a cleanse diet or fad diet to hastily lose weight. It is a controlled method of changing dietary habits in an effort to return to the program prescribed at the time of our weight loss surgery. People do lose weight on the plan because of the dietary changes the plan empowers. This weight loss is considered a sweet bonus, not the primary objective. Please use the plan as a means to lasting weight loss and weight management, not just a quick trick to lose weight. And by the way, losing two pounds in four days is nothing to feel sad about! ***Congratulation!*** You can do this!

Is there a 5DPT for vegetarians?

I have worked on an answer to this question for several years now and have been unsuccessful, which frustrates me because I'm asked this frequently. What I have found is that people who practice a true vegetarian diet do not need the 5DPT because they are living in strict compliance with the vegetarian guidelines and are not likely to have a processed carb snacking habit. People who are (and I mean no offense by this) emotional or political vegetarians are the ones most often asking for a Vegetarian 5DPT. When asked to pinpoint their vegetarian dietary requirements they often say, "Oh, I don't eat anything with eyelashes." That is an emotional dietary parameter. In many cases they have left their dietary choices to emotional chance rather than nutritional sensibility. My advice to these "vegetarians" is to engage in the study of true vegetarian eating and if they so choose deliberately follow that dietary way of life. When the basics of WLS are included with a true vegetarian diet it is unlikely weight gain will result.

You will note there are recipes in the 5DPT that are indicated "vegetarian". That means they meet the standard definition of a vegetarian meal. But it does not imply that there exists a vegetarian 5DPT. Studies suggest a person may live healthy by following a vegetarian diet after weight loss surgery. The trick for vegetarians is to reach the daily requirements of a high protein diet without eating red meat, poultry, fish, or seafood. Of course the first rule of a bariatric diet is "Protein First" in an effort to consume as much as 105 grams of protein a day. The balance of dietary intake should be at least 60 percent protein with the other 40 percent food intake being low glycemic carbohydrates and healthy fats. With the elimination of animal proteins from the diet vegetarians must turn to plant and dairy food for their protein needs. Legumes, low-fat dairy foods, soybeans and soy products, and nuts and seeds are all viable sources of protein for WLS vegetarians. Consider these protein sources in a vegetarian diet:

Legumes: Dried or canned beans such as kidney, cannellini, black beans and navy beans are nutritional powerhouse foods that may be enjoyed daily. One 7-ounce serving of beans provides 15 grams of protein. In addition beans are an excellent source of dietary fiber and they are mineral rich providing B vitamins, iron, zinc, magnesium and phytochemicals. Beans are versatile and can be added to soups, salads, casseroles and stir fries.

Low-fat dairy foods: Dairy foods are another excellent source of protein, but patients of weight loss surgery must eat dairy with caution. Some surgical procedures affect a state of lactose intolerance in patients: it is wise to consult with a bariatric nutritionist if symptoms of lactose intolerance occur. When dairy is tolerated WLS vegetarians can enjoy a 1 cup serving of skim milk, a 6-ounce serving of low-fat yogurt or a 1-ounce serving of low-fat cheddar cheese each providing nearly 10 grams of protein along with calcium and vitamins A, B, and D.

Soybeans and soy products: Soybeans are protein dense: a 7-ounce serving provides 24 grams of protein as well as iron, zinc, vitamin B, and phytochemicals. But Americans have been slow to make soybeans a dietary staple, perhaps because of a few too many tofu-experiments gone badly. New soy-based products take tofu from the strange health food cart to mainstream meals in the form of veggie burgers and veggie tacos. Calcium fortified soy-dairy products, including a variety of milk and cheese items, are commonly available in most supermarkets and make suitable replacements for animal dairy.

Nuts and seeds: A small 1-ounce serving of nuts provides about 5 grams of protein and a rich source of antioxidants including vitamin E and selenium. Nuts are high in fat so the portion must be carefully measured. Under these conditions nuts can provide a healthy snack, or a crunchy topping for salads or desserts.

Weight loss surgery vegetarians must mindfully monitor their dietary intake to ensure adequate protein needs are met. When protein intake is not met weight loss will stall or weight gain may occur. WLS vegetarians should eat a wide variety of protein foods each day to supply their amino acid needs. This can be accomplished by keeping a pantry stocked with legumes, whole grains, nuts and seeds and soy products, and a refrigerator filled with low-fat dairy.

HELP! I am having horrible gas and bloating.

It is quite common for patients of gastric bypass, gastric banding and gastric sleeve weight loss surgery to report an increase in uncomfortable intestinal bloating and the frequent release of foul and offensive gas. Some patients report the problem of gas to be so offensive they suffer chronic embarrassment leading them to isolation. By its nature gastric surgery changes the human digestive process and increases the occurrence of gas. In addition, weight loss surgery patients follow a high protein, low carbohydrate diet which is also known to cause gas. Understanding what causes excessive flatulence is the first step to implementing therapies to reduce the occurrence and offensiveness of this natural body function.

High Protein Diet: Weight loss surgery patients who follow a strict high protein diet frequently report excessive flatulence beyond the 14 releases per day experienced by adults with a healthy digestive tract. In digestion proteins are broken down with the secretion of hydrocholoric acid which allows the activation of pepsin, a protein digesting enzyme. Weight loss surgery patients become deficient in hydrocholoric acid or pancreatin when their intestines are shortened or bypassed with surgery. Therefore the gastric enzymes and acids to facilitate complete digestion are deficient and excessive gas can be produced. A high protein diet, by nature, is a diet low in fiber intake. The absence of adequate fibrous carbohydrates leads to waste material moving too slowly through the large bowel and constipation and flatulence results.

To reduce the occurrence of flatulence associated with a high protein diet stay hydrated by drinking at least 64 ounces of water daily. The water will help to move food along the digestive and intestinal tract preventing the build-up of gas. Eliminate processed meat, cured meat, beans, tofu and soy products from the diet for several days until symptoms of chronic flatulence are reduced.

Sugar Replacers: Weight loss surgery patients are strongly encouraged to eliminate sugar and sweets from their diet. Many people include products labeled "sugar-free" in their diet to satisfy sweet cravings. Sugar-free products use sugar replacers, a term to describe the sugar alcohols such as mannitol, sorbitol, xylitol, maltitol, isomalt, and lactitol, which provide bulk and sweetness to cookies, hard candies, sugarless gums, jams, and jellies. Sugar alcohols evoke a low glycemic response because the body absorbs them slowly making them slow to enter the bloodstream. However, side effects such as gas, abdominal discomfort, and diarrhea, are so extreme that regulations require food labels to state that "excess consumption may have a laxative effect."

To decrease the gas associated with sugar alcohols eliminate or reduce the intake of food containing sugar alcohol. Do not exceed package serving size of sweets made from sugar alcohol.

Therapies to Reduce Offensive Flatulence: The following therapies may be effective in reducing embarrassing and uncomfortable gas and bloating associated with the diet after gastric weight loss surgery

Beano: A few drops help prevent gas formation. Not effective in preventing bloating and gas pain however will prevent gas-passing or flatulence.

Chamomile, ginger and papaya teas: good digestive aides, nerve tonics, and cramp and pain relievers.

Peppermint oil: relieves flatulence and related pain.

How do I define my new normal?

Chapter 7: Day 5 – Solid Proteins

Look where you are! Day 5 & Powerful!

You have made it to Day 5: Congratulations! I hope you are feeling strong and powerful and in charge of your weight loss surgery tool. I knew you could do it and I am proud of you. Today you conclude the test and prepare to embark on Day 6 and the eating plan you will follow consistently to continue losing weight and maintain the healthy weight you desire.

On our final day, Day 5, we introduce solid protein back to our menu. Protein Recommendations: white meat poultry cooked dry and lightly seasoned, beefsteak (if tolerated) grilled or broiled, and anything from Day 3 such as the Breakfast Bakes and anything from Day 4.

Remember to chew-chew-chew. Measure your portion and eat only until you feel your pouch tighten. Please, take only 15 minutes per meal and avoid lingering which eventually leads to a grazing habit. By now you should be out of any carb cycle you were in and perhaps you have lost a pound or two. You have renewed confidence in your pouch and your ability to work the tool for your health and emotional wellness. You did not have the surgery in vain: You still have your tool.

Today, do not go hungry. Remember, you can eat as often as you want provided it is solid protein, consumed without liquids and measured in 4 to 6-ounce portions. Be mindful of the hunger signals your body sends as well as the satiation signals it sends. These signals are your ally in the cause of weight management. Day 5 is not the end of the 5 Day Pouch Test: Day 5 is the beginning of treating your body well and managing your health according to the principles of weight loss surgery. This is the exciting beginning of your new and improved living after weight loss surgery! You Have Arrived!

In the following sub-chapters we will take a look at some of the barriers that get in the way of our best efforts for health and weight management with surgery. Perhaps you have already run into these barriers, most of us have. Keep these solutions in mind next time you hit a road block that threatens to keep you from your goals.

Stop the Comparison!

We live in an intrinsically competitive world. Online communities and the Internet have made it even more so. In our collective quest for better health through weight loss, in our case with weight loss surgery, it is more popular than ever to compare and compete with one another as we pursue personal and highly individualized goals. And while some healthy competition can be a great motivator the comparison of weight loss can lead to utter discouragement.

Contrary to popular culture, weight loss is not a contest. Weight loss is a lifesaving initiative owned by the one taking action.

In online communities I see, even with the 5 Day Pouch Test, that people are making comparisons in how much weight is lost in the 5 days. When they do not measure up to what another person reports losing they consider their own 5DPT effort a failure. It is not.

Unless you pound-for-pound and fork-for-fork competitively gained weight with another person you have no business competing to lose weight. Contrary to popular culture, weight loss is not a contest. Weight loss is a lifesaving initiative owned by the one taking action.

By all means we should compare our experiences. Let's share recipes and exercise tips. Let's give reminders to drink our water and take our supplements. But let's leave the competition to the amateurs. As weight loss surgery patients we understand that our lives were in danger from obesity and we took advanced medical action to change the course. We are much wiser for it.

If you are feeling beaten by the competition I invite you to step back from the scrimmage lines and consider your personal goals and desires. As you own these goals and desires, you also own the pace at which you accomplish these goals. Your worth is not measured against another based on a medical statistic (your weight). Your worth is measured in who you are, a whole person rising above the competition to live your very best life, the way only you know how. The competition is over: let the living begin!

Beyond the Scale: Accepting Healthy Body Weight

In spite of cultural appeal to our vanity the primary reasons for achieving and maintaining a healthy weight should be health and longevity. "Even if our society were to accept fat as beautiful," we read in Understanding Nutrition, "Obesity would still be a major risk factor for several life-threatening diseases. For this reason, the most important criterion for determining how much a person should weigh and how much body fat a person needs is not appearance but good health and longevity." (Whitney & Rolfes, 2005)

Knowing this we can include an acceptance and appreciation of our overall health as part of our weight loss surgery experience and avoid the pitfalls of the single arbitrary finish line we call goal weight. Here are some helpful tips for accepting your healthy body weight:

- Value yourself and others for human attributes other than body weight. Realize that prejudging people by weight is as harmful as prejudging them by race, religion, or gender.
- Use positive, nonjudgmental descriptions of your body.
- Accept positive comments from others. Dismissing a compliment is hurtful to the person giving it and lowers your self-esteem as well.
- Focus on your whole self: your intelligence, social grace, spiritual connections, and professional and scholastic achievements.
- Become physically active, not because it will help you get thin but because it will make you feel good and enhance your health.
- Seek support from loved ones. Tell them of your healthy lifestyle goals and identify how they can support you in your efforts. Connect with others sharing the same goals.

Navigating in the Real World: The Holidays

One of the challenges we face with weight loss surgery is returning to the same environment in which we lived before surgery; the exact environment that contributed to our obesity. The same is true after the 5 Day Pouch Test. So there is no better time than now to look at some of those environmental complications and evolve some strategies to cope with them without giving up our weight management goals. Let's consider the holiday feasting season.

During the feasting season –*Halloween through New Year's Day*-- it is very typical for magazines and news programs to report the calorie count of traditional holiday meals. The Thanksgiving Day Turkey Feast easily comes in at 1,400 calories and the Christmas Day Prime Rib Extravaganza packs in a whopping 1,800 calories. Experts warn us that weight gain from holiday eating is inevitable. But I dare say, it is not the big meals that do us in: it is the BLT's: Bites, Licks, and Tastes. I wish I knew which diet program or person coined the BLT's so I could give them credit, it has been in my diet-talk for as long as I can remember. You have probably heard it too.

It's the BLTs that cause weight gain!

The Bites, Licks, and Tastes will do us more harm than any big meal because even with our little tummy pouches there is always room for another Bite, Lick or Taste. When we sit down to a big meal our pouch fills quickly and when we are full discomfort occurs and further eating adds to that discomfort, so we stop eating. That is how the pouch is supposed to work. But standing in the kitchen stirring a sauce or baking cookies it seems we always have room for little Bites, Licks and Tastes. I've talked to many people who are in the BLT boat with me, maybe you are there too. So here are a few tricks I've learned to help me avoid caloric uptick and weight gain that comes from unchecked BLTs.

Eating vs. Tasting: A skinny professional chef taught me this trick: when preparing sauces, reductions and gravies it is necessary he taste-tests the mixture for seasoning and texture. As a home cook my inclination is to use a soup spoon to take full spoonful of the sauce for my culinary taste-test. "You are using the wrong end of the spoon!" he scolded. The skinny chef demonstrated that by using the handle end of the spoon and just dipping the tip in the gravy for a taste on the tongue he could quickly discern any seasoning adjustments required at the cost of very few calories. "The objective is to taste mindfully and deliberately in order to make an informed decision about the sauce. You, on the other hand," he said, "were eating, not tasting." What an awakening moment! He was correct. In fact, I am certain that in many cases I have eaten a meal's worth of calories in the guise of "testing" while I cook.

You deserve to enjoy the nutritional wellness that can only be achieved by the choices you make with your fork.

Picky Taster: Some things simply do not require a taste test like pasta, rice, potatoes or other starchy side-dishes. Face it: we already know how pasta or rice tastes so when we taste-test pasta or rice we are either tasting to check doneness or we are eating. I realized most of the time my tasting habit is better described as eating. Skinny chef said he learned to test pasta and rice for doneness by taking two samples: one he would chew and the other he would cut with a fork on a cutting board. The simultaneous action of chewing and cutting taught him the feel of doneness with utensils so he no longer needs to taste for doneness. Now he only tests doneness with the fork and cutting board method. As he told me, "I'm in the kitchen for 10 or 12 hours a day. If I tasted a sample from every pot of pasta this kitchen puts out it would add up to hundreds of calories a day eating something that I already know how it tastes. Why take on those calories?"

Spit like a lady. One of the most elegant sophisticated women I know has a job that requires her to taste-test food for a commercial retailer. On a given day she may be required to taste 12 cheesecakes and a dozen different cupcakes. Some job for a person recovering from morbid obesity with weight loss surgery! This classy woman has no qualms about tasting and spitting. She tastes, chews and spits. And then offers her informed, low-calorie opinion on the products at hand. There is no shame in spitting, she has taught me. If you must taste but do not have it in your caloric budget or dietary plan then spit: just spit like a lady and carry-on.

Being in control of your fork always feels better than pie tastes.

Break the sweet-salty cycle. One danger that befalls during the feasting season is indulgent eating that leads to corrective eating. By that I mean indulging in sweet offerings leads us to correct the flavor balance by eating something salty and a cycle of corrective eating begins. Sweet-salty: sweet-salty. Are you familiar with this cycle? It took me a very long time to figure this out and I can recall that as a child my dad would often say he needed something sweet to chase the salty taste away. After gastric surgery this eating cycle can be damaging to our sensitive system throwing our blood glucose levels out of balance, possibly causing dumping syndrome. As well as I understand our nutritional needs following weight loss surgery occasionally I find myself caught-up in this cycle. It happens easily this time of year. Recently I have taken a lesson from the French that for generations have relied upon the palate cleanser between menu courses to remove lingering flavors in the mouth and improve digestion. A palate cleanser effectively stops a sweet-salty cycle of corrective eating. It is a simple and effective fix. Try iced water with a pinch of lemon zest and a squeeze of lemon juice stirred in with a little honey for sweetness. Or try green tea or mint tea, warm or iced, to break an eating cycle.

Awareness is perhaps the greatest weapon we have in the ongoing face of temptation by way of Bites, Licks and Tastes: Awareness that BLTs do contain calories and lead to weight gain; Awareness that weight management for those of us battling morbid obesity is literally a matter of life-and-death; Awareness that we deserve nutritional wellness that can only be achieved by the choices we make with our fork.

Tips to stay on track in the feasting season

Breakfast: Eat a protein breakfast first thing. Use recipes for Day 3 including Breakfast Bakes. A protein dense meal kick starts the metabolism: it also provides a feeling of fullness. Have a second serving of your breakfast bake three hours later to stave hunger while yummy holiday smells fill the air.

Water & Beverages: Drink 24 ounces of water between breakfast and your next meal or snack. A well-hydrated body works efficiently and reduces hunger cravings. Continue to drink water throughout the day: at least 64 ounces. Avoid high-calorie punch or mixed drinks. Drink alcohol only at meals.

If an event is meant to matter emotionally, symbolically, or mystically, food will be close at hand to sanctify and bind it." – Diane Ackerman

Appetizer Buffet: Practice the 2 Bite-1 Bite Rhythm (2B/1B) and liquid restrictions while partaking from the appetizer buffet. Specifically, eat two bites of protein for every bite of fruit or vegetable carbohydrate. If you are eating from the buffet avoid liquids until you have finished your food. Best bet - wait 30 minutes before and after the appetizer buffet for liquids. This is tough in a social setting. If 30 minutes doesn't work in your situation try for a 10 minute pause between eating food and enjoying a beverage.

Slider Foods: Remember that crackers, pretzels, cookies and white breads are non-nutritional slider foods. If you give yourself permission to enjoy some of your favorites remember the liquid restrictions. Following the liquid restrictions will decrease the amount of processed snack foods we eat in a single sitting because there is nothing to wash them down. Even slider foods will help you feel full when observing the liquid restrictions.

The Big Feast: Get greedy with the protein; be stingy with the side dishes. I'm a sucker for the ubiquitous green bean casserole so I'll indulge with a bite or two on a special holiday. Treat yourself to a favorite dish and then let it go. *It is just food.* Remember your liquid restrictions, but celebrate too. It is acceptable to take small sips of your beverage at a big meal. A moist mouth facilitates conversation and surgical weight loss does not exempt us from sharing a conversation and a toast with our loved ones. Give yourself permission to be a participant in this great human experience we call living.

Holiday meals and family gatherings last a few hours; they do not last for weeks. When the meal is over, it is over. Remove your plate and avoid post-meal nibbles during kitchen duty. Better yet, let someone else do clean-up. Go for a long walk: assign kitchen duty to the kid table. Go ahead and say, "My doctor prescribed that I must walk after every meal, I'd love to help but it is important that I take care of my health." Leave the clean-up and the post-meal nibbling temptation to someone else.

Dessert: Contrary to popular belief, food does not have morals. After dinner sweets are neither good nor bad: they are just desserts. If you have a perennial favorite take a bite or two and savor the moment. Then let it go. Discard a too-large serving, this is perfectly appropriate. You may have to be crafty about this to avoid hurting Aunt Edna's feelings, but it is okay to throw away a chunk of pie. Being in control of your fork always feels better than pie tastes.

Kindness: Above all else, *be kind to yourself,* our ongoing theme. Express gratitude for your weight loss tool and for your personal empowerment. Celebrate doing the best you could to find a middle ground to respect yourself and your traditions. In any given week during the Feasting Season you will eat 21 meals. Even the most festive among us is unlikely to enjoy more than six feasting gatherings during that time. That means there are 15 other meal opportunities to get it right. So when a feasting event takes us off plan it is not cause for self-criticism. It is a time for acceptance and moving forward to the next opportunity to nourish our body well.

The day after the feast: Follow the food plan for Day 3. Again, start your day with a protein dense breakfast. Day 3 is a "soft protein" day and the food plan is gentle with your little tummy. Drink lots of water. Avoid slider foods. Take your vitamins and exercise (shopping counts!). Plan your meals and snacks: do not eat leftovers standing at the refrigerator. Pat yourself on the back! You have the power to celebrate a feasting day without allowing it to become the launching pad for a six week downward spiral of unchecked eating that leads to weight gain and poor health.

My feasting season strategies:

- Losing weight is a matter of health: it is not a competitive sport. Contrary to popular culture, weight loss is not a contest. Weight loss is a lifesaving initiative owned by the one taking action. This is your journey: enjoy it at your pace.

- Learn to measure your worth by means other than the bathroom scale. Focus on your whole self: your intelligence, social grace, spiritual connections, and professional and scholastic achievements.

- Develop strategies for navigating in the real world. When we have surgery we changed and then we returned to the exact environment we lived in prior to surgery: the very environment that contributed to our obesity. The only chance we have to make the surgery work is to evolve strategies for navigating our new body in the old waters.

- Always practice kindness. Be kind to yourself, our ongoing theme. Express gratitude for your weight loss tool and for your personal empowerment. Celebrate doing the best you could to find a middle ground to respect yourself and your traditions and your new WLS body. This you deserve.

Day 5 Journal: Solid Proteins

Day 5 concludes your 5DPT. You are now eating solid protein and following the rules and tenets that make weight loss surgery work. Well done! This is the start of your new way of living after weight loss surgery. Keep the enthusiasm alive. You are powerful and you can do this!

Records:	Nutritional Intake – All food and Beverages				
Day/Date: **Weight:**	*Item*	*Pro(g)*	*Fat(g)*	*Carbs(g)*	*Calories*
Water Goal: O O O O O O O O O O Mark 1 bubble for each 8-ounce serving water.					
Vitamins/Supplements:					
Exercise & Fitness:					
Goals/ *Totals:*					
Summary:					

Download 8.5x11" journal at 5DayPouchTest.com – Click Tools
See appendix for journal Days 1-5 for your use.

By Day 5 most of your questions are answered and you have learned a great deal about the 5 Day Pouch Test and why it works. Here are a few of the questions most frequently asked at this point in the plan:

What happens after the 5DPT?

Beginning on Day 6 after the 5DPT we slowly include complex carbohydrate vegetables and fruit in the diet at a ratio of two-thirds protein to one-third complex carbohydrate when measured by volume. We continue to follow the liquid restrictions and avoid slider foods and stay intently focused on the Four Rules. Now that we have recaptured that hell-bent determination that propelled us to have surgery in the first place we use the momentum in our pursuit of a healthy lifestyle and weight management with bariatric surgery.

I did the 5DPT and lost weight, but it didn't stick. Why?

The motivation for doing the 5DPT should always be to get back on track with the WLS dietary guidelines, not to lose weight. That means we take what we learn during the 5 days and apply it to our lifestyle on Day 6 and beyond. If we do the 5DPT simply to knock-off a few pounds and then go back to the very habits that lead to weight regain we will, naturally, regain the weight and then some. When we consented to weight loss surgery we agreed that for the rest of our life we would follow certain dietary guidelines. If we have drifted from the original guidelines the 5DPT can get us back to basics. At that point we must follow the guidelines we agreed to if we wish to sustain weight loss and keep our obesity in remission. Use this as a means to return to following the instructions you were provided by your surgical weight loss center and nutritionist. Go back to doing what worked for you when you were at your best and losing weight or maintaining weight.

What if the 5DPT shows me my pouch is broken?

If you have given the 5DPT your best effort and you still feel like your pouch is not working in the way it was intended to work please see your bariatric surgeon. Several diagnostic tests are available to determine the state of your pouch. In some cases a surgical revision may be necessary due to a pouch failure. Notice it is a pouch failure, not a personal failure when a revision is necessary. Revisions for gastric surgery are common and sadly some needing revisions are made to feel like moral failures when this is not at all the case. A revision is a medical procedure to correct a medical condition. Seek the care of a qualified bariatric team and do what is necessary to protect your health. Please review from Chapter 1, "What you can do if weight regain happens".

How soon can I do the 5DPT again?

Always keep in mind that the 5 Day Pouch Test is to be used a vehicle to get back on track with your WLS basics. It should not be used as a fad diet to quickly knock off a few pounds. Include the 5DPT in your weight management when you do not feel in control of your eating or cravings, when you have strayed from the Four Rules and basic tenets that have worked in the past to help you lose weight, and when you simply need to get back to the basics of WLS. Do the 5DPT when you are in a place mentally to take charge of your health and commit to getting back on track. This gives you the best chance for success. The focus should always be on learning to use the tools that will keep us on track for the long-term.

Can I do the 5DPT every Monday-Friday and then take weekends off?

I hope you won't do this. It takes us back to our pre-surgery diet habits and serves no positive purpose. With surgery it is impossible to put-away the tool for the weekend, so why would we put away our good habits for the weekend? Use the 5 Day Pouch Test as it is designed and move forward with an eye on the long-term goal of better health and weight management making the most of your tool, each day, and every day.

Chapter 8: General FAQ's about the 5DPT

These are general questions about the 5 Day Pouch Test that I have answered many times since the plan was introduced in 2007. You will also find an extensive collection of questions and answers in the monthly 5 Day Pouch Test Bulletins published electronically and delivered by email. Past issues are archived on the website.

5 Day Pouch Test Bulletin – Subscribe at 5DayPouchTest.com

How much weight can I lose?

The 5 Day Pouch Test is not a plan to lose weight, although many people who do the plan report weight loss. When we reach a point where we need to get back to basics with our weight loss surgery the 5DPT is a tool to quickly get us back on track. Closely following the plan helps us break a slider food snacking habit that may have stalled weight loss or caused weight gain. The 5DPT takes our stomach pouch through the dietary progression we followed after surgery with two days of liquid pampering and three days of advancing from soft protein to firm protein to solid protein. During the five days we focus on the Four Rules, especially Protein First. We observe the liquid restrictions and focus on the very reasons we had weight loss surgery in the first place. Most importantly, the 5 Day Pouch Test gives us a renewed sense of confidence in our surgical pouch and our personal power in following a healthy eating plan that supports weight loss and weight maintenance. Any weight loss is incidental to that and should be considered a bonus, not the foremost objective.

Will the 5DPT work for my procedure? (Lap-Band, Sleeve, RnY)

The 5DPT has been successfully completed by men and women with all surgical procedures. All case studies report returning to the high protein, low carbohydrate diet following completion of the test. Gastric bypass patients report the most noticeable tightness in the surgical gastric pouch and in achieving feelings of fullness more quickly. However, adjustable gastric banding (lap-band) patients and gastric sleeve patients report feeling full sooner after doing the 5DPT. People who have done the 5DPT consistently note that returning to liquid restrictions is the single most important action for optimizing the low-volume capacity of their gastric pouch. Again, if you feel you need to get back to the basics of your post-surgical bariatric diet give the 5DPT a try. It is only five days and you may be surprised how powerful you and your pouch are.

I had surgery many years ago. Is it too late for me?

Only you can answer this question. I know of people who had bariatric surgery back in the 1980's --*when the procedure was a simple staple line down the stomach*-- who have successfully done the 5DPT. Many times when people ask me if it is too late to do the 5DPT it is out of fear: fear they will learn their pouch no longer works or fear they will learn the pouch does work. The simple back to basics 5DPT will not cause harm and it is only 5 days of your life. So it is up to you to decide if it is too late.

How soon after surgery can I do the 5DPT?

Without exception patients *must* follow the dietary program directed by their bariatric center for the first year following surgery. No exceptions. I do not recommend or encourage anyone in the first year post-surgery to do the 5DPT. Please, follow the plan your center prescribed specifically for you.

How often can I do the 5DPT?

If a patient is following the program outlined by their center, if they are losing or maintaining weight and feels energized and in control the 5DPT is not needed. It is a specific action to be taken when a patient needs a methodical method for getting back to the basics of post-WLS living. It is not a gimmick or a trick diet; it is a method of taking control when things are out of control. Think of it as your bariatric airbag and hope you never need to use it. But if you do find yourself in peril this airbag is there ready to be deployed. See the FAQ's for Day 5 for more on this topic.

Should I take my vitamins when I'm doing the 5DPT?

Yes, please follow the directions from your doctor or bariatric center and take your vitamin and mineral supplements as prescribed. In addition, take your prescription medications as prescribed. If you have difficulty taking pills without food between meals then take them with a few sips of water about 15 minutes after a meal. Alternatively, try taking them with a mid-morning snack of ½ cup cottage cheese or yogurt. This will help buffer them and prevent the nausea some report when taking vitamins on an empty stomach.

What is a trick to tell me when to stop eating?

As you know, measuring our portions is of first defense to avoid over eating. But as we are living in the real world we know that this is not always possible. Consider these two tricks to help trigger your stop-eating instincts.

First, the fork rule. Even conventional dieters are taught to put down the fork between bites of food, but this is a very difficult habit to acquire. Sometimes it feels like the fork is more an extension of the hand rather than a tool. But by putting down the fork we have time to enjoy the bite in our mouth rather than focusing on loading the fork with the next bite of food. Give it a try the next time you sit down to a meal. I think, like me, you'll find yourself chewing better and enjoying your food more. Digestion begins with chewing so by the time the food reaches the pouch we have put in motion the biological actions that will signal satiation.

One bite under.
Just right,
not too tight.

The next trick I have learned is to stop one bite under full. I call it the "One Bite Under" rule. All my life I've been persuaded by the "food pushers" to have "just one more bite." Before surgery that "just one more bite" contributed to my morbid obesity. After surgery that "just one more bite" has sent me on the run head first to the bathroom more times than I care to admit. Even if I think I can handle or want one more bite, I try to stop short. These days it feels much more comfortable to feel just right rather than too tight. When you find yourself thinking "I'll just have one more bite," put the fork down and think it over for a minute or two. Make an informed choice and stick with it by remembering "Just right, not too tight."

What should I do if carb cravings come back after the 5DPT?

Go Green! Including vegetables in our weight loss surgery diet is not only smart nutrition; it honestly helps tame carbohydrate cravings. Vegetables are complex carbohydrates. They deliver nutrients, minerals, and vitamins to our body and affect blood glucose levels naturally. They give us color and crunch and are willing participants in any preparation from raw and dipped to oven roasted and seasoned with herbs and spices. Remember to follow the 2B/1B rhythm: 2 Bites Protein to 1 Bite Carbohydrate (including vegetable carbohydrate) to keep Protein First in your meal plan. Here are some tips from the USDA for preparing vegetables and enjoying them as part of your healthy plate:

- Buy fresh vegetables in season. They cost less and are likely to be at their peak flavor.
- Stock up on frozen vegetables for quick and easy cooking in the microwave.
- Buy vegetables that are easy to prepare. Pick up pre-washed bags of salad greens and add baby carrots or grape tomatoes for a salad in minutes. Buy packages of veggies such as baby carrots or celery sticks for quick snacks.
- Use a microwave to quickly "zap" vegetables. White or sweet potatoes can be baked quickly this way.
- Vary your veggie choices to keep meals interesting.
- Think soup. Our carb monster soups are perfect year-round for taming the carb-hungry beast within us all.

The rules we signed onto for life.

By and far, the Four Rules are the most universally offered guidelines by bariatric centers for patients of all weight loss surgery procedures. In pre-surgical counseling patients are asked to commit to following the Four Rules as lifestyle habits after surgery. This is an in-depth look at each rule and why it is effective for healthy weight management with surgical intervention. As always, refer to the documentation provided you at the time of your surgery for the specifics advised by your bariatric center.

Rule #1 - Protein First

Regardless of the procedure, patients of stomach reduction surgery for the treatment of morbid obesity are instructed to follow a high protein diet to stimulate healing and promote weight loss. Bariatric centers espouse what is commonly known among weight loss surgery patients as the "Four Rules" the most important of which is "Protein First." That means of all nutrients (protein, carbohydrates, fat and alcohol) the patient is to eat protein first. This is true for all stomach reduction and restriction procedures including gastric bypass, gastric banding (lap-band), and gastric sleeve.

Protein is an essential building block for muscle, blood, skin, hair, and nails. We need it for muscle repair, for building natural immunities, and for proper growth and development. Every cell in the human body depends on it, which is why it is important to get the recommended allowance every day. A high protein diet that is low in carbohydrates and low in fat is believed to promote weight loss due to the metabolic impact of protein. It has the highest thermic effect at 20-30% of all food elements. That means the energy expended during digestion and absorption of protein is 20-30% more than the energy (caloric) content of the food. It takes more energy (calories) to digest and absorb protein than the energy (calories) it contains. In other words, the body must tap into stored energy resources, body fat, to get the job of digestion done. That is why a high protein diet triggers fat loss.

Based on a 1,200 calorie a day diet weight loss surgery patients are counseled by their bariatric nutritionists to eat from 60 to 105 grams of protein a day. This recommendation varies by patient and by nutritionist. For adults without gastric surgery the standard protein intake calculations go like this:

Average protein recommendation:
0.36(g) x body weight (lbs) = grams protein per day

Higher protein recommendation:
0.68 (g) x body weight (lbs) = grams protein per day

Animal products are the most nutrient rich source of protein and include fish, shellfish, poultry and meat. Dairy protein, including eggs, is another excellent source of protein. In fact, the quality of egg protein is so great that scientists typically use eggs as the standard to measure protein quality in other foods. On overage, one ounce of animal or dairy protein contains 6-7 grams of protein as well as many other minerals and vitamins. Nuts and legumes are a fair source of protein but are significantly higher in fat than carefully selected lean animal protein. Also, due to their high fiber content, they may be more difficult for some gastric surgery patients to digest.

For weight loss surgery patients who feel restriction after eating a very small amount of food, protein is not always the most comfortable food choice, particularly lean animal protein. It is essential that gastric weight reduction patients chew their food thoroughly to avoid discomfort when eating. The high protein diet must be sustained even after healthy body weight has been achieved in order to maintain a healthy weight and avoid weight regain. A diet high in protein works to reduce snacking or grazing because protein foods help you feel fuller compared to eating the same amount of starch, sugar, or fat. That satisfied feeling can make it easier to eat fewer calories while you lose weight.

Understanding ketosis in the WLS high protein diet

Often when we hear about a diet that puts the body in a state of ketosis we are fearful having heard that ketosis is a potentially dangerous imbalance of blood glucose, the result of a low carbohydrate, high fat, high protein diet. Ketosis results when the body switches from burning glucose for energy to burning ketones for energy. Glucose comes from carbohydrates which are the body's first choice to metabolize for energy. Ketones are used for energy when there is not enough glucose (from carbohydrates) present in the bloodstream to use for energy.

Clinically stated, "Ketosis is a condition in which levels of ketones (ketone bodies) in the blood are elevated. Ketones are formed when glycogen stores in the liver have run out. The ketones are used for energy. Ketones are small carbon fragments that are fuel created by the breakdown of fat stores. Ketosis is potentially a serious condition if keytone levels go too high." (Whitney & Rolfes, 2005)

Bariatric patients are instructed to follow a high protein, low carbohydrate diet with a modest amount of fat. The body only needs proteins and fats for building and repairing tissue and cells, carbohydrates do not play a part in this metabolic function. Additionally, the body can get all its energy from fats and proteins. A ketogenic diet, which was first developed in the early 1900s, is a high-fat and low-carbohydrate diet. When following a ketogenic diet the body will switch from being a carb-burning machine to a fat-burning machine. As a result weight is lost.

Perhaps the best known ketonic diet is the Atkins plan in which ketosis is deliberately achieved by way of high fat high protein and low carbohydrate diet. According to the Atkins program proper monitoring via urine tests will keep ketosis within safe limits and the dieter can reach an ideal body weight without suffering unbearable hunger. Most weight loss surgery patients are discouraged from following an Atkins-type diet because of the high fat content. Surgery reduces the amount of gastric juice available for digestion and many patients do not tolerate high fat foods.

Speaking to the general population (not necessarily weight loss surgery patients) experts are divided regarding the health risk versus health benefit of a ketogenic diet. Some experts say it is dangerous because if keytone levels are not properly monitored there may be a strain on the kidneys, and a significant loss of calcium excreted through urine may cause kidney stones or osteoporosis. Proponents of a ketogenic diet cite human evolution in their argument saying during most of the time that humans have existed we have been a hunter-gatherer species living in a ketogenic state for extended periods. Documented studies suggest that after a 2 to 4 week period of adaptation human physical endurance is not affected by ketosis. Some studies go so far to suggest that humans do not necessarily need a high carbohydrate intake in order to replace depleted glycogen stores for energy.

We need to work closely with our bariatric center to develop a diet and lifestyle program specific to their condition of obesity and recovery. Ketosis is most likely to occur in the early weeks and months after surgery during the phase of rapid weight loss, and when compliance with the Protein First rule is stringent.

Rule 2: Lots of Water

It isn't breaking news to us that drinking lots of water is part of the post-WLS protocol. We have learned through multiple weight loss attempts that consuming lots of water flushes fat and facilitates weight loss. Especially after WLS drinking lots of water is priority for weight loss and overall good health. In fact, it is so important it is the second of the Four Rules.

Dieters are often told: drink water. Drink a minimum of 64 ounces a day or drink eight glasses of water a day. Weight loss surgery patients don't have a choice: they must drink lots water. Other beverages including coffee, sweet tea, milk, soft drinks and alcohol are discouraged by most bariatric centers and generally do not count toward water intake. Water is the essential fluid for living. Water is one of the most important nutrients the body needs to stay healthy, vibrant, and energetic.

The human body is a magnificent vessel full of water. The brain is more than 75-percent water and 80-percent of blood is water. In fact, water plays a critical role in every system of the human body. Water regulates body temperature, removes wastes, carries nutrients and oxygen to the

Some nutritionists calculate recommended daily water intake based on body weight. Divide body weight by two and drink that many ounces of water a day.

Example for 220 pound person: 220 / 2 = 110

Recommended water intake: *110 fluid ounces per day*

cells, cushions the joints, prevents constipation, flushes toxins from the kidneys and liver, and dissolves vitamins, minerals, and other essential nutrients.

The body will panic if water intake is significantly less than required. Blood cannot flow, waste processes are disrupted, and the electrolytes become imbalanced. Proper hydration prevents inflammation, promotes osmosis, and moistens lung surfaces for gas diffusion. It helps the body regulate temperature, irrigate the cells and organs and promotes all functions of elimination. Certainly by drinking plenty of water many people could resolve inflammation and elimination problems that result from insufficient water intake. Adequate water facilitates weight loss.

Dangers of dehydration

Dehydration is the condition in which body water output exceeds water input meaning we release through elimination and perspiration more fluid than we ingest. Symptoms of dehydration include thirst, dry skin and mucous membranes, rapid heartbeat, low blood pressure and weakness. When a message of thirst is unanswered the symptoms of dehydration may progress rapidly from thirst to weakness, exhaustion, and delirium and end in death of not corrected. Dehydration may easily develop with either water deprivation or excessive water losses.

To avoid dehydration and illness caused by insufficient water balance weight loss surgery patients can take the following measures to ensure adequate water intake:

Lots of Water. Set a daily goal for water consumption and keep track of your intake to make sure you are adequately hydrated. Use a notebook, diet journal or phone app to help you meet your daily water goals.

Fortified Beverages. Vitamin and mineral fortified beverages are beneficial to some weight loss surgery patients. The flavoring makes them more palatable making it easier to consume generous amounts of water. Be certain to enjoy only non-calorie fortified beverages that do not contain sugar or other high calorie sweeteners.

Green Tea or Sun Tea. Freshly brewed green tea or herbal tea served over ice and sweetened with non-calorie sweeteners is another good way to stay hydrated during warm summer weather. The health benefits of green tea and herbal tea may contribute favorably to a well-planned health and weight management program.

Water Containing Foods. Many foods contain a high percentage of water that contributes to body hydration. Enjoy vegetables and fruits such as strawberries, watermelon, lettuce, cabbage, celery, spinach, apples, grapes, citrus, and carrots. All of these foods contain more than 80 percent water which will contribute to hydration and provide a valuable source of vitamins and minerals.

Restrict Liquids, Drink Lots of Water - HUH?

In a country where food and drink go hand in hand weight loss surgery patients are challenged to follow the liquid restrictions as instructed by their bariatric center. But understanding and following the liquid restrictions plays a key role in long-term weight maintenance following gastric bypass, gastric sleeve, or adjustable gastric banding (lap-band) surgeries.

In general, bariatric centers instruct weight loss surgery patients to avoid drinking liquids for thirty minutes before a meal, during the meal, and for thirty minutes following the meal. This easily adds up to 90 minutes of no liquids three times a day: four-and-one-half waking hours. It is easy for patients to become frustrated with these restrictions because another rule of weight loss surgery is to drink lots of water, at least 64 ounces a day. Understanding why the liquid restrictions are necessary and how water intake affects weight management will increase the likelihood a patient will follow the guidelines.

When a person undergoes any of the currently practiced bariatric and metabolic surgeries for weight loss the size of the stomach is reduced significantly to restrict the amount of food which may be eaten at a given time. The size of the restricted pouch varies by procedure, surgeon and patient. What is consistent, however, is that the smaller stomach pouch fills quickly and the patient experiences a feeling of fullness and satiation, which must be sustained following the meal to avoid hunger and cravings later. This is to keep the patient from over eating. In addition, the longer food is kept in the digestive system the more opportunity the body has to absorb and metabolize nutrients. The best way to sustain this fullness is to eat lean protein and low-glycemic complex carbohydrates in a ratio of two bites protein to one bite carbohydrate: the 2B/1B Rhythm.

For many weight loss surgery patients the feeling of tightness or restriction that results following eating is unfamiliar and uncomfortable. In weight loss surgery street talk these patients learn to "eat around the pouch". In many cases that means drinking liquid with solid food which relieves the tightness as the chewed food (chyme: semi-liquid mass of partly digested food) mixes with liquids to form a more fluid liquid slurry which passes through the new stomach outlet more rapidly. The result is increased food intake because patients can eat more food during a planned meal and they are likely to eat again later because they are hungry and the slurry meal failed to satiate hunger for a reasonable amount of time.

As important as it is to follow the liquid restrictions it is equally important to drink adequate water. The body is made up of about 60 percent water. Water assists with the transport of nutrients and waste products throughout the body. Water is present in every process of human biology. Most centers recommend a minimum intake of 64 ounces a day. Others suggest morbidly obese patients drink one ounce of water for every two pounds of body weight.

Organized planning is helpful when following liquid restrictions and drinking lots of water. Begin the day with water and enjoy water between meals, which will also help keep cravings away. Keeping a glass or bottle of water within reach is a steady reminder to sip often and stay hydrated. Newly post-operative patients report drinking tepid or room temperature water is easier on the pouch thus making it possible to drink more.

Rule #3 – No Snacking

Without a doubt, the "No Snacking" rule is the most divisive in the weight loss surgery community. In fact, I've received more angry letters on this topic than any other of the Four Rules. One school of thought is that snacking is absolutely forbidden. The other school swears that three meals plus two snacks a day are essential for the nutritional survival of the weight loss surgery patient.

I am not a doctor and I am not a nutritionist. But I work on the front lines with weight loss surgery patients every day, patients who are many years out from surgery; patients who have lost touch with their bariatric centers. What I do know for certain is this: patients

Ask yourself, "Will what I'm about to put in my mouth contribute to my good health or simply add calories?"

who snack and who are not engaged in extreme athletics gain weight. There is a fine line between snacking intelligently and grazing and few, if any, of us have the self-control to toe the line. In my experience and in my opinion there is no reason for the average person post-WLS to ever engage in snacking. If we follow the high protein diet we will not be hungry in the four to six hours between planned meals; there will not be a blood glucose emergency and there will not be a physiological need to snack.

This may be a very unpopular stand for me to take. But I have spent many years working with my fellow weight loss surgery patients and in every case of weight regain snacking has been involved. And in most cases the initial instructions from the bariatric center were for the patient to eat every three to four hours and somewhere along the third year things went wrong. Snacking on protein bars or nuts became grazing on pretzels and crackers washed down with soda, coffee or tea. Slider foods overruled sensibility.

No Snacking. It is the rule that works.

Now, I'm obligated to tell you to follow the very specific instructions given you by your bariatric center. If they instructed you to have three meals a day and two snacks a day that's fine: please do not feel I'm beating you up here. But please, go get your original notes and detailed instructions. Review the list of approved snacks. Copy that list and post it on your refrigerator to keep your memory refreshed. The snacks your center permitted during the

The most commonly consumed slider foods include pretzels, crackers (saltines, graham, Ritz, etc.) filled cracker snacks such as Ritz Bits, popcorn, cheese snacks (Cheetos) or cheese crackers, tortilla chips with salsa, potato chips, sugar-free cookies, cakes, and candy. You will notice these slider foods are often salty and cause dry mouth so they must be ingested with liquid to be palatable. This is how they become slider foods. They are also, most often, void of nutritional value.

phase of weight loss are the only snacks you are allowed for the rest of your life if you want to maintain your weight loss.

I personally feel the "No Snacking" rule is a tremendous relief. For several years of my adult life, prior to surgery, I had a 40-minute commute to and from work each day. My morbidly obese irrational thinking had me convinced that I could not last that commute without a large soda and giant cookie: both morning and night. Looking back that was about 1,200 calories of snacking I was taking each day just to "survive" my commute. Twelve hundred calories is equal to our full day caloric allowance after surgery! How was it again, that I became morbidly obese? My car was always full of crumbs and the back seat littered with empty cups and cookie wrappers, not to mention the expense of my snacking habit. What a relief when "No Snacking" took that burden from me.

One reason we are prone to break the "No Snacking" rule is because traditional snack foods are ever present in our society and they tend to set more comfortably in our stomach pouch than protein dense food. Have you found yourself able to eat an endless bag of crackers or chips yet struggle to get a few bites of roast chicken down? The crackers are soft and when consumed with liquid create slurry that never compacts in the pouch the way protein does. The cracker slurry slides right through in a steady stream: slider food. Solid protein, on the other hand, settles in the pouch like an unwelcome second cousin on your sofa and lingers just a little too long. So naturally we prefer to eat something that gives us comfort, not discomfort.

But the fact is, the pouch when it is used correctly, is supposed to be a little bit uncomfortable. The discomfort is the signal to stop eating. When we are snacking on slider foods we do not get that signal and we do not stop eating.

Rule #4 – Daily Exercise

The final rule, the one many weight loss surgery post-ops struggle with the most, Daily Exercise. Nothing is more disappointing than hearing a weight loss surgery patient brag that they did not have to exercise to lose weight. It is true; most patients will lose weight without exercise. But patients who do not use the time of rapid weight loss to incorporate exercise into their lifestyle are doing themselves a grave disservice.

Obesity cripples the body. Bone tissues are compromised, joints are swollen, the vascular system is inadequate, and the skeleton overburdened. As weight is lost, the burden on the bones, joints and vascular system is decreased. The body is a magnificent machine. Given proper nutrition and physical motion it will rebuild its broken framework.

The most effective way to heal the body from the ravages of obesity is to exercise. Exercise means moving the body: walking, stretching, bending, inhaling and exhaling. Exercise is the most effective, most enjoyable, most beneficial gift one can receive when recovering from life threatening, crippling morbid obesity. People who successfully maintain their weight exercise daily, not just for weight loss but for life.

How to Increase Activities of Daily Living

We are learning that formal exercise is not always the best or only way to add physical activity to our daily routine. In fact, patients are more likely to become physically active when they gently increase their Activities of Daily Living (ADLs) rather than attempt a full-steam-ahead boot camp-style cardio and strength training regimen from the get-go. The well-known Duke Diet for healthy and lasting weight loss suggests that the first element of fitness is the ADLs which include everything from "waking up, getting out of bed, combing your hair, putting on your robe, stepping out to get the newspaper to doing household chores, taking care of the yard, and walking the dog." According to the Duke Diet program ADLs accumulate throughout the day and burn calories with little or no conscious effort.

Choose activities you enjoy. People stick with exercise when they enjoy it. Choose activities that you look forward to, not dread.

There is never a time following bariatric surgery when it is too late to begin including more motion and activity in our daily routine. Consider these opportunities to increase Activities of Daily Living starting today:

- Do moderate housework like vacuuming and sweeping more frequently and more energetically.
- During TV commercial breaks stand and walk in place, do stretches, knee bends, or arm circles.
- Take the dog for longer, more frequent walks.
- Play actively with children and include brisk walking, bending, tossing or climbing movements at the park or playground.
- Enthusiastically work in the garden mowing the lawn or raking leaves.
- Use stairs instead of elevators or escalators going both up and down.
- Take stretching breaks to loosen tight muscles during long working days at a desk or office job.
- Stand for routine office tasks like sorting paperwork or filing and talking on the phone.
- Do calf raises while standing on line or waiting for the bus.
- Plan hometown walking tours for a leisurely afternoon and explore your neighborhood.

- Bring groceries from the car into the house one bag at a time increasing steps, do arm curls with heavier items such as canned goods before putting away.
- Wash the car by hand instead of going to a drive through car wash. This adds exercise to your day and saves money.

Discover your own opportunities to increase your Activities of Daily Living!

For the best results regular exercise should be part of your 5 Day Pouch Test and a regular part of your *Day 6* and beyond lifestyle. Include at least 30 minutes of exercise every day on most days of the week. A brisk 15-minute walk following each meal is ideal. Intermittent activity throughout the day will increase metabolism and improve blood oxygenation and circulation. Exercise does wonders for your mood. You do not have to run a marathon or bench press a small child. Simply get up, get going, and get moving. Make it a priority to nurture your health and spirit with movement.

Understanding and Avoiding Dumping Syndrome

Dumping syndrome is specific to patients who undergo a malabsorptive bariatric procedure, most commonly gastric bypass. As pre-op gastric bypass patients we are taught to fear the mysterious dumping syndrome and in most cases we are told that avoiding sugar will prevent the occurrence of dumping syndrome. So it comes as a surprise when after having a malabsorptive gastric surgery we experience symptoms that we think are dumping syndrome, yet sugar has not crossed our lips. Most information discussing dumping syndrome following weight loss surgery focuses on avoiding sugar and suggests that some patients experience dumping syndrome while others do not, almost like it were an optional feature of the surgery. Other misinformation suggests that dumping syndrome goes away after time when patients adjust to surgery and eventually they are able to eat sweets.

Very little clinical research is published to help us understand dumping syndrome beyond personal experience. Combine the lack of reputable information with a plethora of urban legend about dumping syndrome and it is easy to understand the confusion.

Dumping syndrome, also called rapid gastric emptying, is defined by the National Digestive Diseases Information Clearinghouse (NDDIC) as, "a condition where ingested foods bypass the stomach too rapidly and enter the small intestine largely undigested. It happens when the upper end of the small intestine, the duodenum, expands too quickly due to the presence of hyperosmolar (substances with increased osmolarity) food from the stomach. "Early" dumping begins concurrently or immediately succeeding a meal." What that means to gastric bypass patients is that food particles are too quickly absorbed by the small intestine because they have gone directly there without the digestive benefits of an intact intestine. The food is literally "dumped" into the small intestine.

To manage this food the pancreas releases excessive amounts of insulin into the bloodstream and the body experiences the symptoms of hypoglycemia. Symptoms may begin immediately or anytime within 3 hours of eating and may include nausea, vomiting, bloating, cramping, diarrhea, dizziness and fatigue. Symptoms do subside as insulin levels return to normal. Many patients experiencing dumping find comfort in lying down or sipping on fortified water or energy drinks served at room temperature.

The medical community generally agrees the treatment of dumping syndrome is through the avoidance of certain foods that cause it. People who have gastric dumping need to eat small meals that are high in lean protein, low in carbohydrates, avoid simple sugars, and should drink liquids between meals, not with meals. The following are three food groups that should be avoided in the treatment and prevention of dumping syndrome in gastric bypass patients:

- **Simple Sugars**: cookies, cakes, candies, bakery items, ice cream, sweet dairy.
- **Simple Carbohydrates**: chips, crackers, processed cereals, pasta with creamy milk sauces.
- **High-Fat Carbohydrates**: French fries, deep fried food, fast food, grilled food with sweet barbecue sauce, cream based soups and sauces.

A diet of carefully chosen lean protein with low glycemic fresh fruits and vegetables is effective in avoiding dumping syndrome. Ongoing research is beginning to implicate hyperinsulinemic hypoglycemia[5] as the cause of rapid

---

[5] Hypoglycemia can occur as a complication of diabetes, as a condition in itself, or in association with other disorders. A person experiencing low blood sugar hypoglycemia may feel weak, drowsy, confused, hungry, and dizzy.

gastric emptying after weight loss surgery but for you and me on the front lines suffering from sweats and chills called dumping, what does that really mean right now? I suggest we become our own personal research scientists and develop a prudent dietary strategy based on current information and personal data that allows us to avoid dumping syndrome and lead a nutritionally balanced life.

Emergency first aid for dumping syndrome

For patients of gastric bypass weight loss surgery an episode of dumping syndrome, or rapid gastric emptying, is physically dramatic and lifestyle disruptive. Prior to surgery patients are instructed to avoid sweet processed carbohydrates, greasy fried food and all simple processed carbohydrates in order to avoid dumping syndrome. Some patients who become lactose intolerant with weight loss surgery experience dumping after eating food that contains lactose: dairy sugar. While most patients comply with dietary guidelines it is inevitable that at some point they will experience a dumping syndrome episode. The following are suggestions for rendering first aid to someone experiencing dumping syndrome. As always, seek emergency care when symptoms persist for an extended period of time.

Provide for Physical Comfort: At the onset of a dumping episode the patient may first notice a sense of disorientation or confusion. This indicates the body is beginning to panic over an excess of insulin flooding the bloodstream. One who has suffered from dumping previously will probably feel a sense of despair as they realize the onset of dumping syndrome. Providing for physical comfort at this time is the first response to a dumping episode. Efforts to interrupt or halt the dumping episode are futile. Many patients of gastric bypass familiar with dumping prefer to isolate from others finding a cool place in which to lie down. Symptoms may include vomiting or diarrhea so patients should find a restful place near a bathroom.

Many will experience a short period of profuse sweating followed by a longer period of chills: providing a blanket is useful to relieve chills. A patient will reach for the blanket when it is needed, the caregiver should not attempt to cover the patient unless asked to do so. The patient may experience

---

Paleness, headache, irritability, trembling, sweating, rapid heartbeat, and a cold, clammy feeling are also signs of low blood sugar.

symptoms of sensory disorder including extreme and abnormal sensitivity light, sound, and touch. These are transient symptoms and many patients find relief when lights are dimmed and they are resting in a reduced-noise environment. Many patients say they prefer not to be comforted by touch from their caregiver because of acute sensitivity to touch during the dumping event.

Hydration and Electrolyte Beverages: Gastric bypass patients who are suffering from dumping syndrome may have been mildly dehydrated prior to the dumping episode. It is important to return the body to a hydrated state by sipping room temperature water or electrolyte fortified sports beverages. Patients should be discouraged from partaking of sugar sweetened beverages or juice in an effort to correct the insulin imbalance. The body is already in a reactionary and corrective state to the insulin surge and efforts to speed-up the correction process are seldom successful.

Seek Emergency Care: Patients should seek emergency medical care when the symptoms of dumping syndrome last for an extended period of time. If a patient loses consciousness immediately seek emergency medical care and provide details for the patient including the bariatric procedure, history of diabetes or hypoglycemia, and an account of food intake prior to the dumping episode.

Not all weight loss surgery patients experience dumping syndrome. It most commonly occurs in patients of malabsorptive procedures, specifically gastric bypass. Patients of adjustable gastric banding (lap-band) and gastric sleeve are not known to have dumping syndrome. Following an episode of dumping patients should consult their bariatric center to identify the cause of the event and make a plan to avoid episodes in the future.

Glycemic Index and the WLS Diet

As we discussed in earlier chapters we have found that including low glycemic fruits and vegetables our high protein diet is an effective way to introduce nutrients and flavor to meals without the negative consequences associated with other high carbohydrate foods. Understanding the Glycemic Index (GI) is the first step to adding nutrients, variety and flavor from vegetables and fruit to the sometimes restrictive diet. But our concerns go beyond the GI number because for some of us even a small amount of high sugar fruit or vegetable eaten without protein or fat may cause immediate glucose response or rapid gastric emptying. We call this dumping syndrome.

Grapes are a good example of a smart food choice that may cause problems catching us off-guard. Grapes have a GI value of 53 ranking them a *LOW* GI Value. That means they have low impact on glucose levels. One cup is considered a serving size. At first glance this would make them a suitable fruit for patients of gastric surgery, but front line research tells us a different story: grapes are beautiful fruit of the Gods just waiting to slip down into our little pouches and morph from healthy fruit snack to spiteful little slider food and dumping disaster.

Here is what happens: We rightly believe grapes are good for us and low calorie, so we do not measure portion size. We enjoy each grape --*which is mostly water and fructose*-- in unmeasured portion as a snack, so there is no buffer to slow the absorption of fructose through the esophagus or intestinal walls of the pouch. We can eat a copious amount of grapes because as fast as we are enjoying them they are sliding right through the stoma. Even with the surgical stomach pouch when eating grapes we never achieve fullness. Unaware of the dramatic glucose load this puts on our body we continue to enjoy our healthy snack when all at once the slam hits us and we are in glucose overload distress: *dumping*. This can happen with any gastric surgery patient who follows a lean protein diet and has developed a low tolerance for glucose surging.

So the short answer, though low glycemic, grapes are a fruit to enjoy with measured caution. As a snack I suggest controlled portions, no more than one cup in a single serving. Make your grape snack a mini-meal and include a one ounce serving of lean meat and one ounce serving of low fat cheese.

Better yet, consider grapes as ingredient food, not just a snack. Here is a classic Southern-Style Chicken Salad that makes wonderful use of grapes in the main dish. The high protein count in the recipe will prevent a glucose overload from the grapes and you get to enjoy a delicious meal.

I just love to share this recipe as an example of how we can enjoy traditional foods in a healthy way while respecting the parameters of our weight loss surgery. And I also love to eat this delicious salad! As you evolve your cooking style seek recipes, like this one, that take a traditional classic and make it work for your needs.

Dressing:
1/4 cup heavy whipping cream
3/4 cup Miracle Whip Light®
1 teaspoon no-sodium all-purpose seasoning blend
Salt & Pepper to Taste

Salad:
2 1/2 cups cooked chicken, chopped and chilled
1 cup celery, chopped
1 cup green seedless grape, sliced
1/2 cup sliced almonds, lightly toasted
4 tablespoons fresh parsley, chopped
Bibb lettuce, leaves separated into six cups , one per serving

For Dressing: In a medium bowl using a whisk whip the whipping cream until fluffy. Fold in Miracle Whip Light®, seasoning blend and season with salt and pepper to taste. Set aside.

For Salad: In a large bowl toss together cooked chopped chicken, chopped celery and sliced grapes. Add dressing and fold together gently until combined. Chill until serving, may be prepared to this stage one day ahead. When ready to serve divide chicken mixture evenly among lettuce cups, garnish with toasted sliced almonds and chopped fresh parsley. Serve chilled.
Nutrition: Serves 6. Each serving provides 363 Calories; 27 grams protein; 24 grams fat; 11 grams carbohydrate.

Chapter 10: Day 6- Beyond the 5DPT

Welcome to your new life: You Have Arrived

Most of us agree that after completing a successful 5 Day Pouch Test the thing we want most is to keep the momentum going. We do not want to have invested time and effort into a five day plan only to return to the behavior and habits that took us off track. Many times I've been asked, "How do I make it stick?" Indeed, I have asked this of myself often. In the LivingAfterWLS Neighborhood we came to call the days and weeks following the 5DPT "Day 6." The name evolved to mean that every day is a new Day 6; a fresh opportunity to use the effective good habits we learned while doing the 5DPT. This chapter is a brief look at Day 6: Beyond the 5 Day Pouch Test.

I love the word diet[6]

Over the years society has whored the word diet until it has become an ugly stepsister loathed by fat and thin alike. In fact, many of us became obese by following the latest "fad diet". You know them all. But did you know that the word diet, a noun, is simply defined as the foods and beverages a person eats and drinks? More historically, diet is a Greek word that means "mode of life," especially one prescribed by a physician that includes the regulation of eating habits. The earliest recorded English definition of diet is "food, daily provisions," and that is the current correct usage.

Yet in our modern civilization we have adulterated the word to mean extreme dietary restriction, odd food combining, punishment, false promises, and fleeting hope. By the time we pursue and undergo weight loss surgery we often declare our emancipation from dieting forever. I know I did. Diets had failed me and I would no longer be in the servitude of the diet industry.

Ten years after weight loss surgery I am not on a diet and I have not returned to dieting servitude. But food, my daily provisions are my diet and to them I am true.

---

[6] Printed with permission from "Day 6: Beyond the 5 Day Pouch Test" by Kaye Bailey, ©2009, 2012 LivingAfterWLS, LLC. All rights reserved.

Let me explain. When I was obese I was either dieting or I was not dieting. The dieting meant I was following a plan, and several times I enjoyed the euphoria of weight loss that others noticed and complimented. But the diets were so oddly structured, as quick-fix diets usually are, that as soon as I stopped following them, and went back to normal, the inescapable weight gain occurred. It was only a few short pounds from euphoria to anguish. This pattern repeated countless times and I learned that dieting does cause weight loss. Not dieting, or going back to normal, causes weight gain.

When I was preparing for weight loss surgery I learned about the Four Rules and, still suffering chronic dieting mentality, believed that I would only need to follow the Four Rules until I achieved goal weight. Then I could get back to normal. At a support group session before having surgery I heard a gastric bypass patient say, "I can eat anything I want, just less of it," with a big hearty belly laugh. Naturally, I assumed this was true, that I would be able to eat anything I wanted and the tool would do the work. I would never ever have to follow a diet again. What a relief.

The truth is, in order to make our tool work we must mindfully follow a diet. Not just during weight loss but for the rest of our lives.

For a long time I thought I was the only one foolish enough to think I would never have to diet again after surgery. But now I know that most of us think we will never have to follow a diet again, surgery will cure us of that.

The truth is, in order to make our tool work we must mindfully follow a diet. Not just during weight loss, but for the rest of our lives.

I ask you to consider your relationship with the word diet. Not long ago I was looking at a road map. The title of the road map was "Geographical Rendering of Highways with Topographical and Historical Features." The word "map" did not appear anywhere on the document. Yet when Jim asked, "May I see the map?" I knew exactly what he was asking for. Map was the best word to describe the tool he wanted to use to make a plan to get from one destination to the next. Sometimes the lowliest word is best.

And so it goes with the word diet. I have been writing about weight loss surgery and dieting for several years. Over that time I have tried to use trendy expressions in lieu of the dreaded D-Word such as way-of-eating, healthy eating, high-protein consumption, WLS-way-of-eating and several others that are just plain silly. So in working on this Day 6 book I was compelled to make amends with our ugly stepsister diet and let her know that we love her for the simple natural beauty she is. We do not despise the ugly whore our society has made her to be.

I offer this, I 🖤 DIET Creed, so we may build a better relationship with food, our daily provisions, and our mode of life:

I 🖤 DIET

Daily adjective: for each day

Intelligent adjective: consistent with reason and intellect: consequent, logical, rational, reasonable

Eating verb: to consume food: to take or have a meal

Triumphs verb: to feel and express uplifting joy over success and victory

Daily Intelligent Eating Triumphs

It turns out our ugly stepsister is a natural beauty of extraordinary simplicity. When you read it like that you just want to make DIET part of your day. It is not the same dirty word nagging easy rapid weight loss from the supermarket tabloids.

Let's discuss each word in our acronym DIET, beyond the definition:

Daily

Perhaps the best known reminder that we must partake food daily is from the Holy Bible, "Give us this day our daily bread." (Matthew 6:11) While that is a prayer of thanks it is also a reminder that to nurture our bodies we must provide food. That means every new day we have the opportunity to make right our nutritional wellness. We have at least three chances daily to feed our body the things it needs so it can give back to us strong bones, healthy lungs, clear eyes, and a sharp mind. How exciting that every single day of our life we have the opportunity to be benevolent to ourselves? I get goose bumps just thinking about my next opportunity to build healthier me.

Intelligent

I love this part of DIET because the weight loss surgery community is notoriously gluttonous for intelligence. Before surgery we are near-hysterical researchers. After surgery we are constant question askers. Why, here you are with this book in hand, seeking intelligence. So of course it stands to reason that when it comes to our DIET we will act with reason and intellect in a consequent, logical, rational, and reasonable manner. Good for you. Our inclination to pursue knowledge and learning is well served by this part of DIET.

We have only covered two of our four words and already you get to treat your body well and behave intelligently every day. I see you smiling. I thought you might grow fond of our new friend DIET.

Eating

Here is another favorite part of this acronym: Eating! Now that we are prepared to make intelligent dietary choices each day we get to the good part, eating. Based on your personal diet prescribed by your bariatric center you may eat three, four, or even five times a day. And since you made intelligent choices you will feel good physically and mentally. Making daily intelligent dietary choices gives us the freedom to enjoy eating without the mental anguish we all feel when we make poor unintelligent dietary choices.

Triumphs

Now for the celebration: You did it! As many times a day as you want you get to feel and express uplifting joy over success and victory! Right now get up off this sofa and you do the best happy dance ever. I'll join you. There is an abundance of joy in your heart: let it out! You have earned this triumph. You are a powerful intelligent individual and you have embraced DIET to make wise and careful choices to bring health and contentment. The health and contentment you deserve to enjoy. Do the happy dance.

No magic tricks: just common sense

Day 6: Beyond the 5 Day Pouch Test is not about magic tricks or secret formulas. It is not a regimented plan of strict do's and don'ts. Day 6 is a common sense approach to making the most of your surgical weight loss tool so that you feel healthy: mentally and physically on most days. It is the act of treating yourself kindly by observing the I 🖤 DIET Creed:

Daily Intelligent Eating Triumphs

Day 6 is liberating, not confining. Following guidelines gives us the choice and opportunity to treat our self well with good nutrition and intelligent choices every day. A well-thought plan will spare us the anguish of poor choices and the unavoidable self-loathing that follows. Nobody goes into weight loss surgery hoping for only a year or two of good results: we want to revel in good health for the rest of our lives. Nobody wants to suffer the disappointment, frustration and embarrassment of weight regain. We do not want to return to suffering the comorbidities of obesity. If I have heard it once I have heard it one-thousand times ten, "Weight loss surgery was my last hope; my final solution."

I 🖤 DIET is a kind-hearted, reasonable, capable and intelligent method of dietary and health management making the most of our surgical weight loss tool. We brought our tool back into the very world in which we became fat armed with Four Rules and a heart full of hope. We knew, by memorization, what we had to do to get through the first weeks and months following surgery. But after that the instructions become vague and we found ourselves wandering, possibly feeling alone. The Four Rules are not enough. They don't address emotional or social issues; they barely give a nod to the physiological issues. And they don't explain well enough why we need to eat protein first or avoid slider foods or why alcohol affects us so differently.

We are very intelligent people: A little more information would have served us well and perhaps helped us avoid some of the struggles. But all is not lost. After doing the 5 Day Pouch Test we have reset ourselves to a newbie-like feeling and here we are at Day 6. We can begin Day 6 with our new knowledge and embrace the I 🖤 DIET.

I believe by now that even those most jaded to the word "diet" will agree I 🖤 DIET is a concept they can embrace. It simply means that we chose daily to make intelligent choices about food; our daily provisions. We have a skeleton plan. We understand the terms of our weight loss surgery: we agreed to them at the time of surgery and surrendering to them is freedom. A consequence of that surrender is independence from obesity; improved health; and emotional freedom from self-loathing. We use knowledge so that we understand what is happening to our bodies and why. We do not relinquish our health to fate because experience has taught us fate is not always on our side.

We take ownership of our medical care by being informed patients asking well-thought questions. We document weights and measurements serving as our own personal statisticians. We provide honest and detailed health histories to our medical team so they can best serve us. When medical complications, such as a revision, occur, we seek understanding and healing. We do not place blame.

Day 6 is a very good place to be.

Five days of eating well

Here you will find all the recipes you need for a delicious and successful 5 Day Pouch Test. These recipes have been tested time and again for their effectiveness in the 5DPT and your gratification both during the plan and for many meals beyond. In addition to enjoying these recipes use them as guides to model your own favorite meals balancing lean protein prepared with fresh healthful complex carbohydrates and controlled amounts of healthy fat.

Avoid substitutions: During the 5DPT please avoid substitutions as much as possible. Each recipe is designed specifically for the designated day of the plan with the amount of protein, carbohydrate, and fat it contains. Changes may decrease the effectiveness of your plan.

Nutritional Analysis: Every effort has been made to check the accuracy of the nutritional information that appears with each recipe. However, because numerous variables account for a wide range of values for certain foods, nutritive analyses in this book should be considered approximate. Different results may be obtained by using different nutrient databases and different brand-name products.

DAYS 1 & 2: Liquids

Days 1 and 2 of the plan are healing days. You treat your pouch like a newborn with gentle protein fortified liquids and soups. Pouch inflammation is reduced and processed carbohydrate cravings subside. Mental focus is on listening to and respecting your body. Your menu on Days 1 and 2 repeats the early days and weeks following bariatric surgery. A diet of simple liquids, including protein drinks, clear broth, creamy soups, and hearty soups takes the guess work out of meal planning so you can focus on making well *and* making right your WLS tool.

All meals on Days 1 and 2 are liquids as defined here. In the 5 Day Pouch Test liquids are defined to include clear broth and creamy soups, protein fortified beverages (protein shakes/smoothies), and hearty soups made of vegetables, legumes with some animal protein and dairy. Please follow the detailed directions for Days 1 and 2 in Chapter 4. Plan your days to include some of these healthful recipes that have been tested and found effective when used as part of your 5 Day Pouch Test. For Days 1 and 2 recipes are divided into sub-categories: *Smoothies & Snacks and Soups.*

Smoothies & Snacks

These smoothie recipes specifically call for UN*JURY*® protein powder: these recipes could easily be called protein shakes or protein meals. I use UN*JURY*® because each scoop has 20 grams of high quality whey protein isolate that is well tolerated by surgical weight loss patients. You can order UN*JURY*® Medical Quality Protein® online at www. UN*JURY*.com. I also use DaVinci Gourmet Sugar Free Syrups to enhance the flavor in my smoothies. You can find DaVinci syrups at many larger supermarkets and online at www.davincigourmet.com. For more sweetness you can add 1 or 2 packets of sugar substitute.

Choco-Mocha Morning Smoothie

Ingredients:
1 scoop UN*JURY*® chocolate protein powder
1 cup skim milk or soy milk
1 tablespoon of decaf instant coffee granules
1 Tablespoon DaVinci chocolate sugar free syrup

Directions: Place all ingredients in the blender and blend until smooth and foamy. *Hint:* If you like an iced smoothie, make ice cubes from brewed coffee and add them to the ingredients as desired. *Nutritionals* will vary depending upon ingredients and products used. Refer to product label to estimate nutritional values.

Vanilla-Berry Smoothie

Ingredients:
½ cup vanilla low-fat yogurt
1 cup skim milk or soy milk
1 scoop UNJURY®Vanilla protein powder
½ cup frozen berries

Directions: Place all ingredients in the blender and blend until smooth and foamy. *Hint:* Fresh fruit may be used in place of frozen and will help reduce the headache that may result from carbohydrate withdrawal. Select fruits and berries from the list of Low Glycemic best choices in Chapter 4: Understanding the Glycemic Index (GI). *Nutritionals* will vary depending upon ingredients and products used. Refer to product label to estimate nutritional values.

Strawberries & White Chocolate Smoothie

Ingredients:
1 cup of water, chilled
1 scoop UNJURY® Strawberry Sorbet protein powder
½ cup frozen strawberries
1 tablespoon DaVinci White Chocolate Sugar Free Syrup

Directions: Place all ingredients in the blender and blend until smooth and frothy. Serve in a chilled glass. *Nutritionals* will vary depending upon ingredients and products used. Refer to product label to estimate nutritional values. *Hint*: Never hesitate to plate and serve your meal beautifully. A well-presented meal enhances the eating experiences and is believed to contribute to prolonged satiety following a meal.

UNJURY High Protein Pudding

Package high protein pudding in single serving containers to grab when a quick snack is required to boost energy and stave off hunger. For on the go meals transport pudding in a cooled lunchbox and serve chilled.

Ingredients:
2 cups cold skim milk or soy milk
2 scoops UNJURY® unflavored protein powder
1 (4-servings) package sugar free instant pudding, any flavor

Directions: In a 2-quart bowl whisk together the cold milk and the protein powder. Whisk in the instant pudding mix, cover and chill. **Nutrition:** Serves 4. Per ½-cup serving: 145 calories, 14 grams protein, 2 grams fat, trace carbohydrate.

High Protein Gelatin

This is the recipe commonly prepared in hospitals for patients recovering from gastric and intestinal surgeries. Many WLS patients continue to include this health-promoting mini-meal in their diet long after healing from surgery.

Ingredients:
1 (4 servings) package sugar free gelatin, any flavor
1/3 cup dried (powdered) egg whites
boiling water and cold water per package directions

Directions: Prepare the sugar-free gelatin according to package directions. When gelatin is dissolved and cold water has been added whisk-in powdered egg whites until completely dissolved. Do not substitute liquid egg whites. Chill until set. Serve cold. For a treat add a 1-tablespoon dollop of fat-free, sugar free non-dairy topping. **Nutrition**: 4 servings. Per serving: 35 calories, 9 grams protein.

Bonus benefit from gelatin

It has long been known that gelatin supports nail and hair growth and that's not just beauty shop gossip. Blame it on those amino acids again! Nails and hair are composed of protein and the amino acids in gelatin provide the building blocks to make them stronger, grow more quickly and reflect your good health with bounce and shine. Adding gelatin to your diet during the first year following weight loss surgery may help to lessen the loss of hair reported by so many bariatric patients. Gelatin is on the approved foods list for all post-surgery dietary stages so give it a chance to love you back. Vegetarians can find plant-based gelatin made of red algae in health food stores.

Powdered eggs and powdered egg whites are fully dehydrated eggs. They are made using spray drying in the same way that powdered milk is made. The major advantages of powdered eggs over fresh eggs are the price, reduced weight per volume of whole egg equivalent, and the shelf life. Other advantages include smaller usage of storage space, and lack of need for refrigeration. Powdered eggs can be used without rehydration when baking, and can be rehydrated to make dishes such as scrambled eggs and omelets.

Powdered eggs are sometimes called dehydrated eggs or meringue powder. Look for them in the baking and cake decorating aisle of your supermarket or craft store. There are also several online sources for powdered eggs offering organic product and other quality features.

Frozen Protein Pudding Pops

These frozen pudding pops are a refreshing treat that can be enjoyed, in moderation, during the 5DPT and the days to follow. Always remember to follow the liquid restrictions when enjoying these treats for a snack or mini-meal.

Ingredients:
2 (11-ounce) ready-to-drink protein drinks, flavor of your choice
1 (4-servings) package sugar-free pudding mix

In a medium bowl whisk together protein drinks and pudding mix. Divide evenly in ice pop molds or small paper cups with wooden sticks or spoons inserted in pudding mix. Freeze until solid. Serve frozen. **Note:** Nutritional information varies by ingredients.

Notes:

Featured here are soup recipes that can be used as your liquid meals for Days 1 and 2 of the 5DPT. Feedback from pouch testers suggests that liquids, such as broth or protein shakes, for some are not satiating and some are struggling to get past the first two days of liquids on the 5 Day Pouch Test. These soups meet the protein requirement, the liquid requirement and they include enough fat and carbohydrate to fuel your body during the pouch test leaving you energized and satiated. In addition, these recipes will help regulate your metabolic hormones: insulin and glucagon, which if you have been in a carb cycle are out of balance.

"Soup is the solvent of memory. For many of us it is love. When I am tired and want comfort, when I want to share happiness, or when I want flavor, my first desire is soup." (Barbara Kafka: Soup: A Way of Life)

You will notice these recipes are slightly higher in fat than our typical recipes from LivingAfterWLS. Humans need dietary fat and use it quite well as fuel. When fat is ingested without being wrapped in white carbohydrates we tend to be self-regulating with our fat intake. After all, have you ever sat down to eat a stick of butter or drink a cup of olive oil? Not too appealing. When you eliminate processed carbs (chips, French fries, doughnuts, cakes, pies, pastries and such), which contain a significant amount of fat, from your diet your body will self-regulate fat intake.

Follow the directions closely: not all soups need to be pureed or blended until smooth. When serving and enjoying soups the most important step is to measure portions, never exceeding 1 cup per serving.

Good idea: Measure soup servings

What I've learned is that soups must be measured. Clear soups or smooth soups without solids should be measured in 1-cup servings and eaten within about 15 minutes. Soups and stews with solids must also be measured, but differently. Use a slotted spoon scoop out solids into a 1/2-cup measuring cup. Put that in your bowl, then add an additional 1/2-cup of the soup - both liquid and solids. This makes a good hearty 1-cup serving that should keep us full and satiated for a long time after the meal. Thick chili with beans and meat is best measured in 2/3-cup servings. It seems like these hearty dishes are much more filling: it is best to start with a smaller portion. Again, with hearty chili and stews avoid exceeding more than 1-cup volume for any meal.

Ham & Cheese Soup

This is a rich creamy soup that pairs the classic flavors of ham and cheese for a delicious meal in a bowl.

Ingredients:
2 tablespoons butter
½ cup carrots, chopped
¼ cup onion, chopped
2 tablespoons flour
1 teaspoon paprika
1 teaspoon dry mustard
6 cups chicken broth, reduced sodium
1 (12-ounce) package processed cheese spread (Velveeta®), reduced-fat, shredded
1 (12-ounce) package light firm silken tofu, diced
2 (5-ounce) cans deviled ham, drained and flaked with a fork
1 cup sour cream, low-fat
salt and pepper, to taste
¼ cup Parmesan cheese, grated
parsley sprigs, for garnish

Directions: In a large Dutch oven over medium heat melt butter. Add carrots and onion and cook and stir until soft and translucent. Stir in flour, paprika and dry mustard using a whisk. Cook for 2 minutes then slowly add the chicken broth whisking to prevent lumps. When soup is thickened add shredded Velveeta®, the diced tofu and ham. Simmer for 20 minutes stirring occasionally. Remove from heat and stir in sour cream. Add salt and pepper to taste and serve garnished with a sprinkle of Parmesan cheese and a sprig of parsley. **Nutrition**: Serves: 10. Per 1-cup serving: 264 calories, 19 grams protein, 15 grams fat and 12 grams carbohydrate.

Note: Substituting other reduced-fat cheese in place of the processed cheese spread will result in a lumpy mixture. Instead, try reduced-fat cream cheese if you prefer it to processed cheese. Do not eliminate the tofu as this vegetarian high protein ingredient is essential to nutritional completeness of this recipe.

This has become an instant favorite for many 5 Day Pouch Test veterans. In place of the pumpkin use a butternut squash puree if you prefer. Canned pumpkin puree is nearly as nutritious as raw pumpkin containing vitamin A, beta carotene and dietary fiber. Pumpkin is a versatile ingredient in soups, casseroles and baked goods that serves our nutritional health well beyond the ubiquitous Thanksgiving pie. Try this soup and keep it in your menu rotation well beyond the 5 Day Pouch Test.

Ingredients:
16 ounces country style sausage*
1 small onion, minced (about ½ cup)
1 clove garlic, minced
1 tablespoon Italian seasoning
1 cup fresh mushrooms, chopped
1 can (15-ounce) pumpkin
5 cups chicken broth, reduced-sodium
½ cup heavy cream
½ cup sour cream
½ cup water

Directions: Over medium heat cook the sausage breaking into small bits. Drain fat. Add the onion, garlic, Italian seasoning, and mushrooms, and cook and stir until vegetables are tender. Add the canned pumpkin, and the broth, stirring well. Cook at a low simmer for 20 to 30 minutes. Remove from heat and stir in heavy cream, sour cream, and water. Serve warm. This soup freezes well in single-serving portions. This soup should not be pureed. **Nutrition**: Serves 8. Per 1-cup serving: 376 calories, 15 grams protein, 32 grams fat, 9 grams carbohydrate.

Country style sausage is bulk ground sausage not in casings. Jimmy Dean® Premium Pork Mild Country Sausage, also called Roll Sausage, is a nationally available country style sausage that works very well in this recipe.

Pumpkin Shrimp Soup

This is another delicious pumpkin soup you will enjoy on Days 1 and 2. Consider stocking-up on canned pumpkin during the fall and winter seasons when it is readily available and priced reasonably. Canned pumpkin can sometimes be difficult to find during the spring and summer.

Ingredients:
2 tablespoons unsalted butter
2 medium onions, sliced
2 medium carrots, sliced
2 medium garlic cloves, minced
1 teaspoon Old Bay Seafood Seasoning®
1 (14-ounce) can fat free reduced sodium chicken broth
1 (15-ounce) can pumpkin puree, no added salt
1 cup whole milk or 1 cup reduced fat evaporated milk
8 ounces cooked shrimp, peeled and deveined (if frozen, thawed)*
freshly grated nutmeg for garnish, optional

Directions: Over medium-high heat in a large soup pot, melt butter and cook the onions, carrots, and garlic, covered until tender, about 10-12 minutes, stirring occasionally. Stir in the Old Bay Seafood Seasoning® and half of the chicken broth. Working in batches puree the cooked vegetables in a blender or food processor following safety guidelines for processing hot food *(see article below)*. Return vegetable puree to cooking pot. Alternatively, use an immersion blender to puree the soup directly in the pot.

To vegetable puree add the remaining broth, pumpkin puree, milk, and thawed drained shrimp. Heat gently to a low simmer, not boiling, continue cooking 5 minutes until soup thickens slightly and is warm throughout. Serve immediately in measured 1 cup portions. Garnish each serving with a sprinkle of freshly grated nutmeg. **Nutrition:** Serves 6. Per 1 cup serving: 245 calories, 19 grams protein, 5 grams fat, 23 grams carbohydrate, 6 grams dietary fiber. **Hint:** For leftovers reheat in the microwave on medium power to avoid overcooking the shrimp.

Substitutions: Canned shrimp, crabmeat, or salmon would work equally well in place of the frozen shrimp if necessary. Be certain you have 8-ounces of seafood solids after draining the liquid. Label weight often includes water weight in canned fish and seafood.

Using the blender to puree soup is a good method for getting a smooth soup as long as certain precautions are followed. Never fill the blender more than half-way and use warm liquids that are well below the boiling point. Most blenders come with a removable stopper on the lid. When blending hot liquids this stopper must be removed and a folded towel can be held in place over the stopper hole. If the stopper is in place steam from the hot liquid creates pressure that literally blasts off the lid creating danger and causing a mess. Blend the mixture with pulses until the desired consistency is reached. Rewarm the pureed soup in the cooking pot.

Lemony Chicken Soup

I found this recipe in Prevention Best Weight Loss Recipes (Anne Rohaiem, 2011) and was intrigued with the inclusion of two eggs at the end of cooking. This method is similar to egg drop soup but I had never considered adding an egg to a more hearty soup. The result is a fresh and light chicken soup with a creamy texture thanks to the addition of eggs. Each 1-cup serving provides 25 grams protein. This soup works well in the 5 Day Pouch Test and will become a Day 6 favorite as well.

Ingredients:
1 teaspoon olive oil
1 small clove garlic, minced
6 cups chicken broth, reduced sodium
1 rib celery, chopped
1 cup shredded carrots
½ teaspoon ground black pepper
¼ teaspoon salt
½ cup orzo* (small-grain pasta)
2½ cups frozen green peas or green beans
3 cups chopped cooked chicken
2 large eggs
3-4 tablespoons freshly squeezed lemon juice (about 1 large lemon)

Directions: Heat olive oil in a Dutch oven over medium heat. Add garlic and cook until light brown, about 1 minute. Add broth, celery, carrots, pepper, and salt and bring to a boil over high heat. Add orzo and reduce heat to a simmer. Cook until orzo is tender, about 8 minutes. Add peas and chicken and simmer 2 minutes. (**Note**: *If freezing portions of this soup do so at this step, before adding eggs. Add eggs to thawed soup in final stage of* *reheating.*) Meanwhile whisk eggs and 3 tablespoons of the lemon juice in medium bowl. Temper egg mixture by slowly whisking in about 1 cup hot broth in a thin stream. Whisk egg mixture into soup and warm briefly over low heat, 2 minutes. Do not boil or eggs will curdle. Adjust seasoning to taste with lemon juice, salt, and pepper and serve. **Nutrition**: Per 1 cup serving: 212 calories, 25 grams protein, 5 grams fat, 16 grams carbohydrate (2 grams dietary fiber).

Note: In Italian orzo means barley, but it's actually tiny, rice-shaped pasta, slightly smaller than a pine nut. Orzo is ideal for soups and wonderful when served as a substitute for rice. Look for orzo in the pasta aisle.

Tomato-Chickpea Soup ~ Vegetarian

One question I answer often is *"Can I have tomato soup on the 5DPT?"* Most tomato soups are heavy with fat and slight on the protein content. However, I recently came across this recipe for Tomato Chickpea Soup and it works well for Days 1 & 2 of the Pouch Test and can also be included in a healthy Day 6 and beyond menu. Not only are the chickpeas nutritionally dense, they are filling and add healthy vegetable protein to the dish. This soup does not have the familiar rich cream texture of traditional soup, but I think you find it quite satisfying. Remember, a serving size is 1 cup. This recipe makes 6 cups so you will have left-overs to enjoy for meals later in the week.

Ingredients:
3 garlic cloves, minced
½ teaspoon red-pepper chili flakes
1 teaspoon ground coriander
3/4 teaspoon coarse salt
1/8 teaspoon caraway seeds
2 tablespoons extra-virgin olive oil
1 (15-ounce) can chickpeas, drained and rinsed
1 (15-ounce) can crushed tomatoes, reduced-sodium
6-ounces roasted red peppers, canned, patted dry, coarsely chopped
3½ cups homemade or reduced-sodium store-bought chicken stock
sour cream for topping

Directions: Using a mortar and pestle or the back of a spoon, crush garlic, chili flakes, coriander, salt, and caraway to form a paste. In a heavy 2-quart saucepan over medium-high heat, heat oil. Add garlic and chili mixture, and cook until just softened, about 3 minutes. Stir in chickpeas, tomatoes, roasted red peppers, and stock. Simmer, stirring often, for 15 minutes. Let cool slightly. Working in batches, puree soup in a blender or use an immersion blender. Rewarm if necessary. Serve with a dollop of sour cream if desired. **Nutrition**: Serves 6. Per 1-cup serving and 1 teaspoon sour cream: 173 calories, 11 grams protein, 8 grams fat (1 saturated), 22 grams carbohydrate

Note: for variety try different canned tomatoes including those flavored with roasted garlic, olive oil, or roasted peppers.

Cream of Turkey Soup

This is a quick and healthy way to use leftover Thanksgiving turkey. Leftover chicken or shredded rotisserie chicken is also good in place of the turkey.

Ingredients:
4 tablespoons (½ stick) unsalted butter
1 large onion, chopped
10 ounces cooked turkey, finely shredded (discard skin)
2½ cups chicken stock
1 tablespoon fresh tarragon
½ cup heavy cream

Directions: Melt the butter in a large, heavy bottom pan, then add the onion and cook for 3 minutes. Add the turkey to the pan with 1½ cups of the chicken stock. Bring to a boil, then let simmer for 20 minutes. Remove the pan from the heat and let cool. Transfer the soup to a food processor or blender and process until smooth. Add the remainder of the stock and season to taste with salt and pepper. Garnish with the tarragon and add a swirl of heavy cream. Serve warm. **Nutrition**: Serves 4. Per serving: 342 calories, 18 grams protein, 28 grams fat, 4 grams carbohydrate.

The Joy of Soup:

It is not very often that I hear from someone who struggles with technical issues when eating soup after weight loss surgery. Soup doesn't get "stuck" going down and if we eat too much the discomfort is short-lived (compared to eating too much solid food that is poorly chewed and eaten quickly). In fact, when post-WLS patients discover soup it often becomes their go-to comfort food. When animal protein is cooked into a soup it is moist and succulent making it easy to chew, swallow, and digest. Cooked vegetables are more readily tolerated by many WLSers compared to raw vegetables. And grains like pearl barley or quinoa are portion controlled and digestible when included as an ingredient in soup. Perhaps it sounds cliché but there is truly joy in a simple healthy cup of soup.

Stock your freezer: Soups, stocks, and broths are easy to freeze. Use heavy-duty freezer bags or plastic containers, but be sure to leave some room for expansion as the liquids freeze. Identify the contents in writing, and be sure to mark down a use-by date (in general, three months). You can also freeze stock and broth in an ice cube tray and then transfer to freezer bags or plastic containers. When you're ready to use the cubes, melt them with boiling water.

Ham & Split Pea Soup

Split peas are a widely popular legume available year-round throughout the United States. They are an abundant source of fiber and protein and also supply a good amount of minerals including potassium, and the disease fighting B-vitamin, folate. A mild sausage compliments the flavor of split pea soup, but for a spicier soup select a hot sausage. Consider garnishing with sour cream to add richness and dairy protein.

Ingredients:
8 slices bacon or 8 ounces bulk pork sausage
½ medium white or yellow onion, chopped
1 cup carrot, chopped
1 pound dry green split peas
16 ounces chicken broth
2 cups water
1 cup ham cubes
1 each bay leaf
ground pepper, to taste
¼ teaspoon nutmeg, freshly grated

Directions: In a large heavy Dutch oven cook the bacon or sausage over moderate heat, stirring until crisp. Transfer to paper towels to drain. Leave rendered bacon fat in pot and cook the onion and carrots until translucent and soft. Add remaining ingredients and bring to a simmer. Simmer uncovered, stirring occasionally for two hours. Add more water if soup is too thick for your taste. The soup should be dense in order to leave you feeling full longer. Discard bay leaf and serve warm topped with crumbled bacon.
Nutrition: Serves: 12. Per 1-cup serving: 184 calories; 13 grams protein, 4 grams fat, 25 grams carbohydrate, 10 grams dietary fiber.

For our purposes with the 5DPT some recipes are sub-titled vegetarian. By definition these are lacto ovo vegetarian recipes. According to Suzanne Havala, M.S., R.D. in *Being Vegetarian for Dummies*, "A lacto ovo vegetarian diet excludes meat, fish, and poultry but includes dairy products and eggs. Most vegetarians in the U.S., Canada, and Western Europe fall into this category. Lacto ovo vegetarians eat such foods as cheese, ice cream, yogurt, milk, and eggs, as well as foods made with these ingredients." (Suzanne Havala, 2001) Please consider this definition when selecting recipes from LivingAfterWLS publications to support a vegetarian diet.

Black Bean Soup ~ Vegetarian

Beans are naturally a low-glycemic food and one of nature's nutritional power packs. They are considered good sources of protein, fiber, B vitamins, iron, zinc and magnesium.

Ingredients:
1 cup dry black beans
olive oil spray
½ cup diced onion
½ cup diced celery
½ cup diced carrot
1 large red pepper, roasted
1 tablespoon minced fresh garlic
2 quarts vegetable broth
¼ teaspoon ground cumin
½ teaspoon salt
1 teaspoon chopped fresh oregano
2 teaspoons chopped fresh parsley
2 teaspoons chopped fresh cilantro

Directions: In a large bowl, cover black beans with 4 cups of water and soak overnight. Rinse beans in a colander with fresh water and drain. Lightly spray a large saucepan with olive oil spray. Over medium-high heat cook and stir onion, celery, carrot, roasted pepper, and garlic Add vegetable broth and black beans. Bring to a boil, reduce heat, and simmer for 1 hour. When beans are tender, pour into a food processor and puree. Add cumin, salt, oregano, parsley, and cilantro. **Nutrition**: Serves 6. Per 1-cup serving: 140 calories, 13 grams protein, 27 grams carbohydrate, 5 grams dietary fiber.

Both lentils and barely are low-glycemic, and each with their distinctive flavors, contribute to make this zesty, satisfying winter soup a meal in itself. The turmeric and curry powder lend an exotic flavor.

Ingredients:
1 tablespoon oil
1 large onion, finely chopped
2 cloves garlic, crushed or 2 teaspoons minced garlic
½ teaspoon turmeric
2 teaspoons curry powder
½ teaspoon ground cumin
1 teaspoon red pepper flakes
6 cups water
1½ cups vegetable or chicken stock
1 cup red lentils
½ cup pearl barley
1 (15-ounce) can crushed tomatoes
salt and pepper to taste
fresh parsley, chopped, for garnish

Directions: Heat the oil in a 3-quart saucepan. Add the onion, cover and cook gently for about 10 minutes or until beginning to brown, stirring frequently. Add garlic, turmeric, curry powder, ground cumin, and red pepper flakes, and cook, stirring, for 1 minute. Stir in the water, stock, lentils, barley, tomatoes, and salt and pepper to taste. Bring to a boil, cover and simmer about 45 minutes or until the lentils and barley are tender. Serve sprinkled with parsley or coriander. **Nutrition**: Per 1 cup serving: 180 calories, 12 grams protein, 5 grams fat, 25 grams carbohydrate.

Hot & Sour Soup ~ Vegetarian

This vegetarian soup provides ample protein with the inclusion of tofu. Be sure to stir fry the tofu cubes as directed for the best flavor.

Ingredients:
2 medium red chilies, coarsely chopped
6 tablespoons rice vinegar
5 cups vegetable broth
2 stalks lemon grass, halved
4 tablespoons soy sauce, reduced-sodium
1 tablespoon sugar

½ lime, juiced
2 tablespoons peanut oil
1 package (16 ounces) firm tofu, cubed
4 ounces mushrooms, sliced
4 medium scallions, chopped
1 cup bok choy, shredded

Mix the chilies and vinegar together in a small non-reactive bowl. Cover and let stand at room temperature for 1 hour. Meanwhile, bring the vegetable broth to a boil in a 3-quart saucepan. Add the lemon grass, soy sauce, sugar, and lime juice, then reduce the heat and simmer for 20-30 minutes. Heat the oil in a preheated wok; add the tofu cubes and stir-fry over high heat for 2 to 3-minutes, or until browned all over. (You may need to do this in 2 batches, depending on the size of the wok.) Remove with a slotted spoon and drain on paper towels. Add the vinegar-chili mixture, mushrooms, tofu cubes, and half the scallions to the stock mixture and cook for 10 minutes. Mix the remaining scallions with the bok choy and use to garnish the soup before serving. **Nutrition**: Serves 6. Per 1-cup serving: 269 calories, 13 grams protein, 11 grams fat, 33 grams carbohydrate.

DAY 3: Soft Protein

As on Days 1 and 2, for the next three days you get to eat as much as you want as often as you want. But there is a catch: you must follow the plan. Again there are specific menu choices for Day 3. Today we introduce soft protein served in carefully measured portions. After two days of 5DPT liquids the introduction of soft protein is a welcome dietary change. It is likely on Day 3 you will start to feel that "newbie" tightness in your pouch. In addition, your hunger or carb cravings are likely to be diminished. Continue to observe the liquid restrictions and take your meals only on a "dry" pouch. Your dry pouch will hold soft protein longer prolonging feelings of satiety.

Protein Recommendations Day 3: canned fish (tuna or salmon) mixed with lemon and seasoned with salt and pepper, eggs cooked as desired seasoned with salt pepper and/or salsa, fresh soft fish (tilapia, sole, orange roughy), baked or grilled, and lightly seasoned. Yogurt and cottage cheese are allowed in ½-cup servings, and 1-ounce cheese servings, such as string cheese, are an acceptable between-meal snack provided liquid restrictions are followed. Vegetarian animal protein replacement products such as tofu or vegetable and legume patties are acceptable on Day 3.

Please follow the detailed directions for Day 3 in Chapter 5. Plan your days to include some of these healthful recipes that have been tested and found effective when used as part of your 5 Day Pouch Test. Our Day 3 recipes are divided into sub-categories: *Eggs & Bakes and Fish and Seafood Soft Protein.*

Eggs & Bakes

According to the American Egg Board, energy boosting foods are in demand. An egg, nature's answer to the quest for a near-perfect protein, is also your answer to the quest for a highly available, highly functional protein ingredient. Consider the facts:

Eggs contain the most easily digestible, most readily available protein compared to any other type.

Eggs are used as the standard for measuring the protein quality of other ingredients.

Processed eggs contribute the same high-quality protein as fresh.

These recipes take advantage of the protein value and nutritional benefits of eggs. In general, eggs are well-tolerated after gastric surgery and readily metabolized into energy and tissue building protein. Consider eggs for any meal of the day.

Hard-Cooked Eggs

As instructed by the American Egg Board: Place as many eggs as desired in a single layer in a saucepan. Add enough water to come at least 1 inch above the eggs. Cover saucepan and place on high heat, and bring water to a boil. As soon as the water begins to boil turn off heat and remove saucepan from stove. Keep the saucepan covered and let eggs sit in the hot water for 12 to 15-minutes. When time is up run cold water over eggs to cool them. To remove shell, crackle it by tapping gently all over. Roll egg between hands to loosen shell. Peel the eggs starting at the large end. Hold egg under running cold water or dip in bowl of water to help ease off shell.

Any time we eat it should be with the intention of providing our body nutritious food that it can digest and absorb in order to efficiently and powerfully fuel the metabolic process of living.

One egg provides 6 grams of protein, or 12% of the Recommended Daily Value (RDV) based on a 2000 calorie a day diet. Eggs provide the highest quality protein found in any food because they contain all of the essential amino acids our bodies need in a near-perfect pattern. While many people think the egg white has all the protein, the yolk actually provides nearly half of it.

The high-quality protein in eggs helps you to feel full longer and stay energized, which contributes to maintaining a healthy weight. In fact, research[7] shows that eggs eaten at the start of the day can reduce daily calorie intake, prevent snacking between meals and keep you satisfied on those busy days when mealtime is delayed. Research indicates that high-quality protein may help active adults build muscle strength and middle-aged and aging adults prevent muscle loss. Consuming eggs following exercise is a great way to get the most benefits from exercise by encouraging muscle tissue repair and growth.

---

[7] American Egg Board: Incredible Edible Egg® http://www.aeb.org/

Start your morning with this Mock Breakfast Burrito and you will have energy to burn. You may not be able to hold this full serving, so refrigerate leftovers for a snack if you get hungry later in the day

Ingredients:
2 eggs or ½ cup egg substitute
cooking spray
1 ounce Cheddar cheese, shredded
2 tablespoons refried beans
1 tablespoon salsa

Directions: Measure the refried beans onto your plate and heat until warm in microwave. Set aside. Spray an 8-inch skillet with cooking spray and scramble eggs or egg substitute to desired doneness adding cheese in the last minute of cooking. Top heated beans with egg mixture and salsa. **Nutrition**: Serves 1. Per serving: 174 calories, 13 grams protein, 9 grams fat, 2 grams dietary fiber.

Mocha Peanut Butter Bites

Stir these together in a medium bowl and divide into 8 equal portions. Wrap each portion separately for a single serving. They are sure to cure your peanut butter blues.

Ingredients:
1 (single serving) package instant high protein oatmeal
4 scoops UN*JURY*® chocolate protein powder
1 tablespoon flax seeds, ground
1/3 cup peanut butter, unsalted
¼ to ½ cup soy milk*

With a spatula or wooden spoon blend all ingredients, adjusting the amount of soy milk to reach your desired consistency. **Nutrition**: Serves 8. Per serving: 141 calories, 14 grams protein, 6 grams fat, 8 grams carbohydrate.

Note: Look for instant high protein oatmeal similar to Kashi® Go Lean Instant Oatmeal, available in most markets. If you prefer substitute reduced-fat evaporated milk for the soy milk.

These hearty dishes are intended to energize your day from the very first bite. Breakfast bakes are high in protein, crazy good with flavor and easy to prepare and serve. Take the time to start your day with one of these dishes, which will satiate hunger and fuel your activities. Please note: nutritional information is for a normal (FDA guidelines) serving size. It is expected that a weight loss surgery patient will eat only enough to fill their small stomach, which should be considerably less than a normal sized serving. Leftovers make great lunch selections to be quickly reheated in the office microwave oven.

Bacon Swiss Squares

Traditional pork bacon is very good in this recipe. Use turkey bacon or vegetarian soy bacon in place of the pork bacon if you prefer; follow the same directions.

Ingredients:
2 cups biscuit baking mix (Bisquick®)
½ cup cold water
non-fat butter flavor cooking spray
8 ounces Swiss cheese, sliced
1 pound bacon, cooked and drained, chopped
4 whole eggs
4 egg whites
¼ cup milk
½ teaspoon onion powder (not onion salt)

Preheat the oven to 425°F. In a large bowl, combine the baking mix and water; stir 20 strokes. Turn onto a surface dusted with baking mix; knead 10 times. Spray a 13x9x2-inch baking dish with cooking spray. Press the dough into the bottom of the baking dish. Arrange cheese over dough. Sprinkle evenly with cooked chopped bacon. In a large bowl, whisk eggs, egg whites, milk and onion powder; pour over bacon. Bake on a lower rack in the preheated oven for 15 to 18-minutes, or until a knife inserted near the center comes out clean. Cut into 12 equal pieces and serve immediately. Serves 12. Per serving: 372 calories, 18 grams protein, 27 grams fat, 14 grams carbohydrate.

Soggy crust: a soggy crust can be the result of high atmospheric humidity or higher moisture content in the eggs and other ingredients. To avoid soggy crust pre-bake the crust for 6 to 8 minutes in the preheated oven before topping with cheese, bacon, egg mixture. After topping the crust return the Bacon Swiss Squares to the oven and continue to bake 12-16 minutes until eggs are set and cooked through.

Spinach-Sausage Egg Bake

Spinach is a nutritional powerhouse loaded with beta carotene, folate, vitamin C, and the phytochemical lutein, which helps maintain vision. Surprisingly, spinach is also a good source of vegetable protein. Most WLS patients report good digestibility of spinach, particular cooked spinach as in this recipe that uses frozen chopped spinach that has been thawed and squeezed dry.

Ingredients:
1 pound country style sausage
1 small onion, chopped
cooking spray
1 (7-ounce) jar roasted red pepper, drained and chopped
1 (10-ounce) package frozen chopped spinach, thawed, squeezed dry
1 cup all-purpose flour
¼ cup Parmesan cheese, grated
1 teaspoon dried basil
½ teaspoon salt
8 large eggs
2 cups milk, 2% low-fat
1 cup provolone cheese, shredded

Directions: Preheat oven to 425°F. Coat a 3-quart baking dish with cooking spray, set aside. In a 10-inch skillet, cook sausage and onion over medium heat until meat is no longer pink; drain. Transfer to the prepared baking dish. Sprinkle with half of the red peppers; top with spinach. In a large bowl, combine the flour, Parmesan cheese, basil and salt. In another bowl whisk eggs and milk; stir into flour mixture until blended, but still lumpy. Pour over spinach. Bake, uncovered, for 15 to 20-minutes or until a knife inserted near the center comes out clean. Remove from oven, top with provolone cheese and remaining red peppers. Return to oven and bake 3 to 5 minutes or until cheese is melted. Let stand for 5 minutes before serving. **Nutrition**: Serves 6. Per serving: 638 calories, 30 grams protein, 45 grams fat, 27 grams carbohydrate. Very good served microwave warmed for lunch the following day.

This recipe makes a generous casserole perfect for family brunch or potluck gatherings. It holds well on a buffet table and may be served at room temperature.

Ingredients:
2 tablespoons butter
2 cups Cheddar cheese, shredded
2 cups cooked ham, cubed
12 large eggs
½ cup evaporated milk
2 teaspoons prepared mustard
salt and pepper, to taste

Directions: Drizzle butter into a 3-quart baking dish. Sprinkle with cheese and ham. In a mixing bowl, beat the eggs, evaporated milk, mustard, salt and pepper. Pour over ham and cheese. Bake uncovered, at 350°F for 40 to 45 minutes. Let stand for 5 to 10 minutes before serving. **Nutrition**: Serves 8. Per serving: 324 calories, 23 grams protein, 24 grams fat, 4 grams carbohydrate.

Puffy Turkey & Swiss Omelet

This quick omelet is a great breakfast, lunch, snack, or dinner for Day 3 of the pouch test. It is particularly appealing on Day 3 because the fluffy texture of the eggs is gentle on your freshly pampered pouch. I like to use the pre-cooked Jennie-O® Oven Roasted Premium Portion Turkey Breast.

Ingredients:
butter-flavor cooking spray
¼ cup onion, finely chopped
½ cup cooked turkey breast, chopped
2 large egg whites (or equivalent egg white substitute)
¾ cup egg substitute
2 tablespoons water
salt and pepper to taste
1/3 cup Swiss cheese, reduced-fat, shredded

Coat a 10-inch nonstick omelet pan or skillet with cooking spray; place over medium-high heat until hot. Add onion, cook and stir until tender. Add chopped turkey, and cook and stir until warm. Slide to a small plate and tent with foil to keep warm. You will use this mixture to top the omelet in the final step.

In a medium bowl using an electric mixer beat egg whites at high speed until stiff peaks form (do not overbeat). In another large bowl whisk together the ¾-cup egg substitute, water, salt and pepper. Fold in the fluffy beaten egg white into egg substitute mixture.

Wipe the skillet clean with paper towels and coat with cooking spray. Place over medium heat until hot. Spread egg mixture in pan. Cover and reduce heat to low. Cook, covered for 5 minutes until puffy. Increase the heat to medium, uncover, and cook 3 minutes longer or until golden on bottom. Watch closely. Slide omelet to a serving plate, spread the turkey and onion mixture evenly on top and top with Swiss cheese. *(If you like, slide the omelet under a preheated broiler to melt cheese)*. Slice into four equal portions. Serve warm. After the leftovers have cooled wrap in plastic or parchment paper and store refrigerated. Reheat gently in the microwave oven or enjoy at room temperature as a snack or meal. The leftover omelet is delicious with slices of fresh vine-ripe tomatoes. **Nutrition**: 4 Servings. Per serving: 88 calories, 12 grams protein, 3 grams fat, 3 grams carbohydrate.

Notes:

As a rule on Day 3 fish is the preferred menu option because it is softer and moister than canned poultry. In addition, fish canned in water is considered low fat, a direction we are heading during the 5DPT. However, the chicken and poultry will take on a softer texture when prepared according to the recipes provided and it will work in much the same way as canned fish. For example, the Parmesan-Tuna Patties are a fan favorite. People with an aversion to fish have enjoyed this recipe substituting canned chicken or canned turkey for the tuna.

Parmesan Tuna Patties

By and far this is **the** favorite recipe of the 5 Day Pouch Test. In fact, after serving this recipe to the people at your table you can expect to have it requested over and over again. Tuna is an outstanding source of lean protein at 27 grams per 4 ounce serving. Tuna also provides good amounts of healthful omega-3 fatty acids which contribute to healthy circulation and heart health.

Ingredients:
1 (6 ounce) can albacore tuna, in water
1 tablespoon mayonnaise
1 large egg
2 tablespoons Parmesan cheese
2 tablespoons ground flax meal
1 dash garlic powder
1 dash onion powder
1 tablespoon olive oil

Directions: Drain tuna. Blend all ingredients in a medium size bowl and form into patties. Heat 1 olive oil in shallow skillet over medium-high. Fry patties in hot oil (I use olive oil, but cooking spray also works well) until brown on edges. Turn and continue to cook until done. **Nutrition**: Recipe makes 4 patties. Each tuna patty provides 132 calories, 16 grams protein, 7 grams fat, 2 grams carbohydrate.

Note: Flax meal, made of ground flaxseed, is rich in omega-3 fatty acids which appear to help lower the risk of heart disease. Flaxseed adds a mild nutty flavor to foods and should be included regularly in a healthy diet. Weight loss surgery patients should use ground flax meal rather than flaxseed for ease of digestion.

Fish Cakes

While a bit more time consuming than using canned fish, fresh fish also prepares well into cakes and offers greater variety to keep your menu interesting. This recipe uses fish fillets that are quickly poached. The cakes are light and the citrus brightens the flavor with a hint of sweetness.

Ingredients:

1 pound firm fish fillets, cut into large chunks
½ teaspoon salt
¼ cup + 2 tablespoons 2% Greek yogurt
¼ cup chopped fresh parsley
1 egg yolk, beaten
1 tablespoon Dijon-style mustard
1 tablespoon freshly squeezed lemon juice (from 1/2 lemon)
¾ cup plus 2 tablespoons panko or bread crumbs (divided)
3 green onions, white parts minced
¼ teaspoon freshly ground black pepper
¼ cup canola oil
low-fat tartar sauce, optional

Directions: Steam fish: Put about an inch of water in bottom of large nonstick skillet and bring to a simmer over medium-high heat. Season fish with ¼ teaspoon of the salt and add it to the pan. Cover pan and simmer fish over low heat until just done, 6 to 8 minutes. Remove from pan with slotted spoon and drain on paper towels. Pour out the water and dry pan. Allow fish to cool slightly, about 5 minutes, and pat completely dry.

Flake fish in medium bowl with forks or your fingers, removing any bones as you go. Add yogurt, parsley, egg yolk, mustard, lemon juice, 6 tablespoons of the panko, scallions, pepper, and remaining 1/4 teaspoon salt. Stir to combine. Shape mixture into eight round cakes; coat cakes with remaining ½ cup panko and shake off the excess.

Heat 2 tablespoons of the oil in the nonstick skillet over medium heat. Add fish cakes and cook until brown and crisp, 2 to 3 minutes. Add the remaining 2 tablespoons oil, turn cakes, and cook until golden brown on the other side, 2 to 3 minutes longer. Drain on paper towels. Serve hot with a low-fat tartar sauce, if desired. *Nutrition*: Serves 4; 2 fish patties per serving. Per serving: 291 calories, 29 grams protein, 14 grams fat, 12 grams carbohydrate.

Like other cold water fish salmon is an excellent source of omega-3 fatty acids. In addition, canned salmon is a terrific source of calcium that is readily absorbed. A 3-ounce serving of canned salmon provides 17 grams of protein along with vitamins B6 and B12 and niacin.

Ingredients:
1 (14.75 ounce) can salmon with liquid, flaked
1 slice of bread, shredded
3 tablespoon chopped green onion, including the green parts
1 tablespoon fresh chopped dill weed, or 1 teaspoon dried
1 egg
½ teaspoon sweet paprika
salt and pepper to taste
1 tablespoon canola oil

In a large bowl, gently mix together the salmon, bread, green onion, dill, egg, paprika, salt and pepper. Form into 8 patties; each about 1/2 inch thick. Heat oil over medium high heat in a 10-inch skillet. Cook the patties until nicely browned on both sides, about 3 to 4 minutes per side. **Nutrition**: Serves 4. Per serving (2 patties): 213 calories, 23 grams protein, 11 grams fat, 4 grams carbohydrate.

Salmon and Black Bean Patties

Increase the amount of dietary fiber you eat by including black beans in recipes. This salmon patty is enhanced with black beans. Serve your favorite tomato salsa on the side.

Ingredients:
1 (7.5-ounce) can pink salmon, drained
½ cup canned black beans, rinsed and drained
¼ cup dry bread crumbs
¼ cup sliced green onions
1 egg white
1 tablespoon lime juice
¼ teaspoon seafood seasoning
salt and pepper to taste
1 tablespoon canola oil

Place salmon in a medium bowl and break with fork. Add beans, bread crumbs, green onions, egg white, lime juice and seasonings. Stir gently to combine. Shape mixture into four 1-inch thick patties. Refrigerate for 30 minutes or until ready to cook, no longer than 24 hours. Heat oil in a large skillet over medium heat: cook patties 2 to 3 minutes per side or until firm and brown. Serve warm with tomato salsa. Nutrition: Serves 2, 2 patties each. Per serving, 308 calories, 18 grams protein, 15 grams fat, 19 grams carbohydrate.

Shopping Hint: Select cod, halibut, tilapia or other firm textured white fish. Thaw frozen fish. I prefer to use thawed tilapia fillets because they are of firm texture, mild flavor, and affordable. Select a firm white fish that is free of bones and skins. Be sure to safely thaw frozen fish fillets following package instructions.

To-Go: Cranberry Turkey Roll-Ups

This is a terrific recipe to use on Day 3 and a great method to keep in mind when preparing portable meals to support your weight loss surgery diet. Experiment with different meats, cheese and condiments to add variety and interest to portable meals.

Ingredients:
1 pound deli-style turkey, reduced-sodium, sliced
4 ounces cream cheese spread with chives and onions
2 tablespoons cranberry sauce, no-sugar-added

Directions: Place two slices of turkey on a cutting board and spread with 1 teaspoon of cream cheese spread, and 1 teaspoon of cranberry sauce. Roll tightly, and secure with a toothpick and place in refrigerator container. Repeat with remaining ingredients, and cover tightly with plastic wrap. *Nutrition*: Serves 4. Per serving: 232 calories, 27 grams protein, 10 grams fat, 5 grams carbohydrate.

DAY 4: Firm Protein

Look where you are: Day 4! Way to Go! You have the most difficult part of the 5 Day Pouch Test behind you and now is the time to start focusing on what you have learned and how you will use your new knowledge to eat and live well beyond the 5DPT. Remember we signed up for life when we had weight loss surgery: today is a new chance to make right our commitment for better health and weight management using the tool and our personal power. *You Can Do This!*

Protein Recommendations: ground meat (beef, poultry, lamb, game) cooked dry and lightly seasoned; shellfish, scallops, lobster, steamed and seasoned with citrus, herbs and vegetables; salmon, or halibut steaks, grilled and lightly seasoned. Vegetarian products including tofu and vegetable burgers are acceptable.

By now you should be experiencing that familiar tightness that will reassure you that your pouch is working. Remember to drink plenty of water between meals. Take some time to meditate and rediscover the wonder of your pouch. Please follow the detailed directions for Day 4 in Chapter 6. Plan your days to include some of these healthful recipes that have been tested and found effective when used as part of your 5 Day Pouch Test. Our Day 4 recipes feature firm protein fish, shellfish, seafood, ground poultry and meat prepared with fresh herbs, vegetables and fruit for your culinary enjoyment. Day 4 recipes are organized in two categories: *Fish and Seafood and Ground Poultry and Meat.*

Fish and Seafood

Our global marketplace has made fish and seafood accessible and affordable. Salmon, tuna, and meaty fish such as swordfish, monkfish, and halibut are available fresh at most supermarkets. Along with plenty of high-quality protein, these lean satisfying fish supply B vitamins, potassium, and moderate amounts of omega-3 fatty acids. Consider including fish in your diet at least once a week to take advantage of the health supporting nutrients in your high protein diet. The fish and seafood recipes here are effective during the 5DPT on Day 4 and work well for your WLS and family menu beyond the Pouch Test.

Greek Halibut with Feta-Spinach Topping

The mild taste of halibut lends itself well to Greek seasoning and pungent feta cheese. Green spinach and red tomatoes make this dish visually appealing and rich in heart healthy phytochemicals. A small portion, served at room temperature, is a pleasing lunch. Other fish can be used for this recipe. At the market select seasonally fresh fish on the day it will be prepared.

Ingredients:
4 (4-ounce) halibut fillets
2 teaspoons Greek seasoning, salt free
cooking spray
1 (10-ounce) package frozen chopped spinach, thawed and squeezed dry
1 plum tomato, coarsely chopped
¼ cup basil and tomato flavored feta cheese, crumbled

Season the halibut fillets evenly with the Greek seasoning. Coat a 10-inch skillet with cooking spray and heat over medium-high heat until hot. Add fish and cook 4 to 5 minutes, turn all fillets. Remove skillet from heat. Evenly divide the spinach, tomato and feta atop the fillets. Return skillet to heat, cover, and cook 4 minutes longer until spinach is hot, cheese has started to melt, and fish flakes easily when tested with a fork. Serve warm. **Nutrition**: Serves 4. Per serving: 147 calories, 25 grams protein, 3 grams fat, 4 grams carbohydrate, 2 grams dietary fiber.

Sunflower Orange Roughy

Orange roughy is a relatively large deep sea fish with a firm flesh of mild flavor. It is sold skinned and filleted, fresh or frozen. This crispy-on-the-outside, tender-on-the-inside baked fish is flavorful and satisfying while being protein dense. The inclusion of corn flake crumbs adds crunch without turning this into a carb-heavy recipe. Other soft fish may be used in place of the orange roughy. This is a good reheated lunch on Day 5.

Ingredients:
¼ cup corn flake crumbs
2 tablespoons dry roasted sunflower kernels
1 teaspoon salt-free all-purpose seasoning blend
4 (4-ounce) orange roughy fillets
1 tablespoon lemon juice
cooking spray

Directions: Preheat oven to 425°F. On a piece of waxed paper combine the corn flake crumbs, sunflower kernels, and seasoning blend. Place orange roughy fillets on a plate and sprinkle with lemon juice. Dip fillets in corn flake mixture and press crumbs to adhere to fish. Place on a foil-lined baking sheet lightly sprayed with cooking spray. Use any remaining crumb mixture to press on fish. Bake the fish on the middle rack in a preheated oven for 10 to 12 minutes or until fish is done. Serve warm. *Nutrition:* Serves 4. Per serving: 201 calories, 23 grams protein, 9 grams fat, 6 grams carbohydrate. *Note:* Sunflower seeds are a nutritional power ingredient packed with vitamin E and folate. They also provide goodly amounts of the minerals magnesium, copper, iron, and zinc.

Salmon with Mustard Cream Sauce

Salmon is rich in omega-3 fatty acids which appear to have several health benefits including lowering triglycerides, maintaining heart rhythm, and decreasing the risk of clot formation in the arteries. Once you have completed the 5DPT consider including salmon in your menu at least once a week to take advantage of the health promoting nutrients it provides.

Ingredients:
4 (4 to 6-ounce) skinless salmon fillets
cooking spray
black pepper
½ cup sour cream, reduced-fat
1½ tablespoons Dijon-style mustard
2 teaspoons fresh dill, chopped
1½ teaspoons lemon juice
1 clove garlic, minced
¼ teaspoon salt

Directions: Preheat broiler and spray broiler pan lightly with cooking spray. Place salmon fillets on a broiler pan, and spray them lightly with cooking spray, season with black pepper. Broil 8 to 10-minutes or until salmon flakes when tested with a fork. *Sauce:* Meanwhile, in a small bowl combine sour cream, Dijon-style mustard, fresh dill, ¼ teaspoon black pepper, lemon juice, garlic, and salt. Place one filet on each plate and garnish with 2 tablespoons of the Mustard Cream Sauce. Serve warm, 1 fillet per person, with 2 tablespoons of sauce. *Nutrition:* Serves 4 (1 fillet and 2 tablespoons sauce). Per serving: 254 calories, 36 grams protein, 10 grams fat, 3 grams carbohydrate.

Orange Glazed Salmon

This succulent salmon includes freshly squeezed orange juice and fresh orange slices. I have found that when we include a sweet taste with a firm protein, such as orange and salmon, our after dinner sweet cravings are diminished.

Ingredients:
4 (4 to 6-ounce) salmon fillets
salt and pepper to taste
cooking spray
3 tablespoons soy sauce, reduced-sodium
1 orange, zest grated and reserved, juiced
2 oranges, sliced

Directions: Season salmon fillets to taste with salt and pepper. Coat a 10-inch skillet with cooking spray, heat over medium-high. Add salmon and cook 4 to 6 minutes per side until fish is done. Remove to a plate and tent loosely with foil. Return skillet to pan, add orange juice, orange zest, and soy sauce. Increase heat to high and stir and cook for 1-minute to deglaze the pan and slightly reduce the sauce. Place each salmon fillet on a plate, top with 1 tablespoon of sauce and serve warm with orange slices. **Nutrition**: Serves 4. Per serving: 148 calories, 23 grams protein, 4 grams fat, 1 gram carbohydrate. **Note**: If you plan to use the leftovers for a future meal, refrigerate the cooked salmon and the sauce separately. Reheat leftovers gently in the microwave to avoid over cooking.

Parmesan Baked Fish

This mayonnaise-Parmesan topping is great on baked firm-flesh fish of all kinds. Use frozen fish fillets that have been thawed per package directions, or select the freshest fillet from your fish market on the day the recipe will be prepared. This is a fantastic dish and method to include on your Day 6 and beyond menu.

Ingredients:
¼ cup low-fat mayonnaise or salad dressing
2 tablespoons grated Parmesan cheese
1 tablespoon snipped fresh chives or sliced green onion
1 teaspoon Worcestershire sauce
cooking spray
4 (4 to 6-ounce) fresh or frozen and thawed skinless fish fillets

Directions: **Sauce.** In a small bowl stir together mayonnaise, Parmesan cheese, chives, and Worcestershire sauce. Set aside. **Baked Fish.** Preheat oven to 450°F degrees. Rinse fish; pat dry with paper towels. Place fish in a 2-quart square or rectangular baking dish coated with cooking spray. Spread mayonnaise mixture evenly over fish. Bake, uncovered, in preheated oven for 12 to 15-minutes, or until fish flakes easily when tested with a fork. **Nutrition:** 145 calories, 21 grams protein, 6 grams fat, 1 gram carbohydrate. Nutrition based on average cold-water fish; refer to package labeling for nutritional data specific to your ingredients.

Sesame Tuna

Sesame seed has a nutty, slightly sweet flavor that makes it versatile enough for use in baked goods such as breads, pastries, cakes, and cookies as well as an interesting ingredient for savory dishes. History tells us this is the earliest known seasoning. The addition of sesame seeds to protein creates a nutty flavor and texture improving the enjoyment of the meal. Find sesame seeds in the spice aisle. Sesame seeds turn rancid quickly because of their natural oils: pay close attention to the expiration date and taste before adding to a recipe to ensure freshness. After opening store sesame seeds refrigerated.

Ingredients:
½ teaspoon salt
4 (4 to 6-ounce) tuna steaks
2 tablespoons sesame seeds
2 teaspoons sesame oil
12 green onion tops, cut into 2-inch strips
1 tablespoon soy sauce, reduced-sodium

Directions: Season tuna steaks with salt, and then sprinkle sesame seeds on both sides of each steak pressing gently into fish. Heat the sesame oil in a 12-inch skillet over medium-high heat. Add tuna, and cook for 2 to 4 minutes on each side or until fish flakes easily when tested with a fork. Remove from pan to serving platter, and tent loosely with foil to keep warm. Add green onions and soy sauce to pan, and cook and stir for 3 minutes until green onions are tender. Divide evenly over tuna fillets. Serve warm, 1 fillet per serving. **Nutrition:** Serves 4. Per serving: 249 calories, 41 grams protein, 6 grams fat, 5 grams carbohydrate. **Note:** substitute canola oil for the sesame oil if desired.

The fat content is higher in this recipe because of the 5 grams of monounsaturated from the avocado. Monounsaturated fats are known to help reduce the levels of LDL (*the bad*) cholesterol. In addition, the richness of the avocado is particularly satiating, and tends to reduce post-meal hunger cravings.

Ingredients:
4 (4 to 6-ounce) tuna steaks
Mrs. Dash® Garlic & Herb Seasoning Blend, to taste
1 tablespoon olive oil
1 cup salsa
1 avocado cut in 8 slices

Directions: Season tuna steaks to taste with the garlic and herb seasoning blend. In a 10-inch skillet heat the olive oil over medium-high heat until hot. Add tuna steaks and cook 3 to 4 minutes on each side until done. In the meantime, warm the salsa in the microwave oven. Serve each tuna steak topped with ¼ cup of salsa and two slices avocado. **Nutrition**: Serves 4. Per serving: 188 calories, 27 grams protein, 13 grams fat, 6 grams carbohydrate. **Note**: the tuna steaks may also be cooked on an outdoor gas or charcoal grill over medium-high direct heat.

Buttery Lemon Shrimp

This is a healthy take on the classic shrimp scampi. Reheat leftovers gently for an enjoyable afternoon snack or toss with scrambled eggs for a protein dense breakfast on Days 4 and 5 and Beyond the 5DPT.

Ingredients:
zest of 1 lemon
1 tablespoon fresh chives, chopped
¼ cup yogurt-based spread (see note)
2 tablespoons lemon juice
1 teaspoon Worcestershire sauce
½ teaspoon paprika
1 tablespoon olive oil
1 pound peeled and deveined large shrimp
1 teaspoon Old Bay® Seafood Seasoning

Directions: Combine lemon zest with chopped chives and set aside. In a small bowl mix the yogurt-based spread, lemon juice, Worcestershire sauce, and paprika. Set aside. Place the olive oil in a 10-inch skillet over medium heat. Add the shrimp and Old Bay® Seafood Seasoning and cook and stir until shrimp turns pink. Add the yogurt spread and continue cooking until shrimp are done. Divide shrimp and sauce evenly among four bowls and garnish with the lemon zest and chives. **Nutrition**: Serves 4. Per serving: 171 calories, 26 grams protein, 6 grams fat, trace of carbohydrate. **Note**: At our home we love the healthy and readily-available yogurt-based spread Brummel & Brown. It is heat stable and has a creamy buttery taste. Brummel & Brown is 35% vegetable oil and 10% non-fat yogurt. It is made in the USA by Unilever.

Spicy Stir-Fry Shrimp

This is a quick and easy recipe that can be adapted for Day 6 and beyond by adding your favorite blend of stir-fry vegetables to the bell pepper, celery, and green onions.

Ingredients:
1 tablespoon canola oil
1 red bell pepper, sliced into thin strips
1 rib celery, sliced diagonally into ½ inch pieces
4 green onions, sliced diagonally into ½ inch pieces
1 teaspoon Mrs. Dash® Extra Spicy Seasoning Blend (more to taste)
1/3 cup chicken broth, reduced-sodium
1 pound large shrimp, peeled and deveined

In a large (12-inch) skillet or wok heat the canola oil to very hot. Add bell pepper strips, celery slices, and green onions. Cook and stir until vegetables are just tender. Add spicy seasoning blend and chicken broth, stir to combine. Add the shrimp, continue stirring and cooking over high heat until shrimp turn pink and are opaque in the center. Serve warm. **Nutrition**: Serves 4. Per serving: 178 calories, 29 grams protein, 5 grams fat, 4 grams carbohydrate.

Citrus Bay Scallops

Bay scallops are generally harvested only on the East Coast but are widely available in the United States, fresh and frozen. They are small: the muscle is about ½-inch in diameter. The meat of the bay scallop is sweeter and more succulent than that of the larger sea scallop. They cook quickly; watch closely to avoid over-cooking.

Ingredients:
1 tablespoon olive oil
1 pounds bay scallops
2 tablespoons lemon juice
1 tablespoon chopped fresh parsley, plus sprigs for garnish
1 teaspoon grated orange zest
2 cloves garlic, minced (optional)
salt and pepper to taste

Directions: In a 10-inch skillet set on medium-high, heat the olive oil. While it heats in a medium bowl toss together the bay scallops, lemon juice, chopped parsley, orange zest, and minced garlic. When oil is hot add scallop mixture and cook and stir until scallops are done. Season with salt and pepper to taste, and garnish with parsley sprigs. Serve warm. **Nutrition**: Serves 4. Per serving: 185 calories, 29 grams protein, 5 grams fat, 5 grams carbohydrate. **Note**: Serve the leftovers, chilled, over mixed greens with light citrus vinaigrette. This makes a healthy, portable, and tasty Day 6 lunch.

Pan-Seared Scallops with Cherry Tomatoes

Sea scallops are about 1½ inches in diameter. The meat is chewy, sweet, and moist. They must be cooked quickly to avoid becoming rubbery. In addition to pan searing they are used in soups, stews, and salads. This recipe requires quick cooking over very high heat. A 3-ounce serving of sea scallops is only 75 calories and contains 14 grams protein with only trace amounts of fat and carbohydrate.

Ingredients:
1-pound sea scallops, fresh (or frozen and thawed)
1 tablespoon olive oil
1 (8-ounce) package cherry tomatoes
2 tablespoons balsamic vinegar
2 tablespoons fresh basil, chopped

Directions: Heat the olive oil in a 10-inch heavy-bottom skillet over high heat. When the oil is hot add the scallops and allow them to sear and cook quickly, do not disturb or the flesh will tear. As the scallops become opaque, carefully turn and cook another 2 to 3 minutes until done. Remove to a plate and tent loosely with foil to keep warm. Lower heat to medium-high, and add cherry tomatoes to skillet. Cook and stir until tomato skins just begin to pop. Stir in balsamic vinegar and fresh basil, and cook another minute, stirring to coat all tomatoes. Serve warm tomatoes, with scallops, drizzling with the balsamic vinegar pan sauce. **Nutrition**: Serves 4. Per serving: 123 calories, 20 grams protein, 1 gram fat, 7 grams carbohydrate.

Ground meat and poultry

Ground meat and poultry are affordable and readily available in most markets. Many weight loss surgery patients who include lean ground meat and poultry in their diet report good digestibility and satiation. In addition, meals made with ground meat and poultry can be shared among family and friends without complaints about *diet* food. Try these recipes and experiment to make them your own for Day 4 of the 5 Day Pouch Test and many meals beyond.

Turkey-Parmesan-Pesto Meatballs

These meatballs come together quickly and have a rich flavor from the pesto sauce. The onion helps keep the lean meat moist. They are good broken and included in scrambled eggs for breakfast on Day 5. Pesto is an uncooked sauce made with fresh basil, garlic, pine nuts, parmesan or Pecorino cheese and olive oil. The ingredients can either be crushed with mortar and pestle or finely chopped with a food processor. This classic, fresh-tasting sauce originated in Genoa, Italy. There are many finely crafted artisan pesto sauces available today at supermarkets and farmer's markets.

Ingredients:
1½ pounds ground turkey, white meat only
¼ cup pesto sauce
1/3 cup Parmesan cheese, grated
1 small white onion, finely chopped
½ teaspoon salt
additional pesto for dipping

Directions: Preheat oven to 375°F. In large bowl, gently combine ground turkey, ¼ cup pesto, Parmesan cheese, onion and salt. Shape mixture into 30 equal meatballs. Place meatballs on a wire rack above a foil-lined rimmed baking sheet. Make sure they are not touching. Bake in the preheated oven for 15 to 20-minutes. Serve warm with additional pesto sauce for dipping. **Nutrition**: Serves 6. Per (5-meatball) serving: 202 calories, 31 grams protein, 7 grams fat, 2 grams carbohydrate.

Slow Cooker Thai Peanut Meatballs

This convenient slow cooker recipe cooks in just 2 hours on high heat. With only three convenient ingredients it makes the grade for a terrific weeknight family friendly meal. For Day 4 enjoy 2 to 4 meatballs: stop eating at the first sign of fullness. For the family and meals beyond the 5DPT serve the meatballs with rice and stir-fried vegetables for a balanced meal.

Ingredients:
1 (13.5-ounce) can coconut milk
1 (3.5-ounce) box A Taste of Thai® Peanut Sauce Mix (both inner envelopes)
1 (16-ounce) package frozen beef meatballs
sliced green onion and lime wedges for garnish

Directions: In the bowl of the crockpot whisk together the coconut milk and peanut sauce mix. Add the frozen meatballs and stir until all meatballs are coated with the sauce. Cover and cook on high for 2 hours, stirring once during cooking. Serve warm drizzled with sauce. **Nutrition**: Serves 4. Per (4 meatball) serving: 350 calories, 18 grams protein, 22 grams fat, 14 grams carbohydrate.

Veggie Mushroom-Swiss Patty Melts

For vegetarians who eat dairy products *(lacto ovo vegetarians)* this is a delicious and satiating Day 4 recipe that can be made ahead and reheated in the microwave for an easy meal. Consider Veggie Mushroom-Swiss Patty Melts for your portable and filling Day 5 lunch.

Ingredients:
4 (2.8 ounce) frozen vegetarian burger (such as Boca Burger®)
¼ cup chicken stock, reduced-sodium
1 (8 ounce) package sliced mushrooms
1 small onion, chopped
black pepper, to taste
cooking spray
4 (1 ounce) slices Swiss cheese, reduced-fat

Directions: Preheat oven broiler. In a 10-inch skillet cook veggie burgers according to package directions. Set aside and keep warm. In the same cooking pan, heat the chicken stock, scraping any browned bits from the pan. Add the mushrooms, and onion, and cook and stir over medium-high heat until the vegetables are tender. On a foil lined cookie sheet sprayed with cooking spray place the four veggie patties and divide the mushroom mixture evenly on top of each burger. Place one slice of Swiss cheese on each burger. Place under broiler to melt cheese. Watch closely to avoid burning. Serve warm. **Nutrition**: Serves 4. Per serving: 162 calories, 23 grams protein, 5 grams fat, 9 grams carbohydrate. **Note**: You may also use this recipe preparation using ground meat or poultry.

Classic Salisbury Steak

Classic comfort food, Salisbury steak is traditionally a ground beef patty flavored with minced onion and seasonings before being fried or broiled. It was named after a 19th-century English physician, Dr. J. H. Salisbury, who recommended that his patients eat plenty of beef for all manner of ailments. Salisbury steak is often served with gravy made from pan drippings. To suit our different tastes this recipe may be prepared with ground beef, pork or white meat poultry.

Ingredients:
1 pound ground meat of your choice
1/3 cup dry breadcrumbs
½ teaspoon salt
¼ teaspoon pepper
1 egg
1 large onion, sliced
1 can (14.5 ounces) condensed beef broth
1 can (4 ounces) mushrooms, drained
cooking spray
2 tablespoons cold water
2 teaspoons cornstarch

Directions: Mix ground meat, breadcrumbs, salt, pepper and egg: shape into four equal size patties. Over medium-high heat, cook patties in 10-inch skillet sprayed with cooking spray. Turn patties occasionally cooking until brown, about 10 to 12 minutes. Remove to a plate and tent loosely with foil to keep warm. Drain excess fat from skillet. Add onion, broth, and mushrooms, cook and stir to bring browned bits up from pan. In a small bowl whisk together water and cornstarch, then whisk cornstarch mixture into onion mixture, still cooking over medium-high heat. Return patties to pan and simmer about 10-minutes until sauce reduces, and meat patties are cooked and tender. Serve meat patties with ¼ cup of sauce per serving.

Note: Below nutrition data is provided for ground beef, pork, and white meat poultry: 1 meat patty with ¼ cup sauce.

Per serving using extra lean ground beef: 321 calories, 27 grams protein, 21 grams fat, 6 grams carbohydrate and 1 gram dietary fiber.

Per serving using lean ground pork: 354 calories, 24 grams protein, 25 grams fat, 6 grams carbohydrate and 1 gram dietary fiber.

Per serving using ground white meat poultry: 225 calories, 25 grams protein, 11 grams fat, 6 grams carbohydrate and 1 gram dietary fiber.

Notes:

DAY 5: Solid Protein

Day 5 and you did it! I knew you could. This is your final day of the 5DPT and your re-entry into the healthy way of eating that will allow you to lose or maintain weight, manage your blood sugar, and simply feel good: isn't that the ultimate goal? Protein choices include poultry, beef, pork and anything from Day 4. Here are several dinner recipes you can enjoy on Day 5 and beyond. Bring forward some breakfast ideas from Day 3 and lunch ideas from Day 4 for a full day of chewing, eating, satiety, and loving that sweet little working pouch of yours.

Chipotle-Jalapeno Chicken with Black Beans

This flavorful chicken and bean recipe comes together quickly for an easy weeknight meal on Day 5. The added fiber from the beans is filling and nutritious.

Ingredients:
1 tablespoon Mrs. Dash® Southwest Chipotle Seasoning Blend
4 (4-ounce) chicken breasts halves, skinless, boneless
cooking spray
½ cup Monterey Jack cheese with jalapeno peppers, shredded
2 tablespoons canned jalapeno peppers, diced
1 (15-ounce) can black beans, rinsed and drained
¼ cup mild salsa

Directions: Season both sides of the chicken pieces with the Southwest Chipotle Seasoning. Coat a 12-inch skillet with cooking spray and place over high heat. When heated add chicken to pan, and cook 7 to 10-minutes on each side until done. While the chicken cooks, put beans and salsa in a medium sized microwave safe bowl and heat on high power 3 to 4-minutes, until warm, stirring once. Remove chicken from heat; sprinkle with cheese. Cover to allow cheese to melt and serve garnished with sliced jalapenos. **Nutrition**: Serves 4. Per serving: 282 calories, 35 grams protein, 8 grams fat, 15 grams carbohydrate, and 6 grams dietary fiber.

Mustard Baked Chicken

This is an easy baked dish that is good for cooler evenings. If you prefer use ready-to-cook boneless skinless chicken pieces in place of the bone-in fryer chicken pieces. It may also be prepared in a slow cooker using frozen chicken pieces and cooking on high 2 to 4-hours or low 4 to 6-hours.

Ingredients:
1 (2½ to 3½ lbs.) broiler-fryer chicken, cut up
cooking spray
1/3 cup brown mustard
1 tablespoon cooking oil
1 tablespoon soy sauce, reduced sodium
2 teaspoons heat-stable granular sugar substitute

Directions: Preheat oven to 425°F. If desired, remove skin from chicken. Place chicken in a 3-quart rectangular baking dish coated with cooking spray. Bake in a preheated oven for 15 minutes. Meanwhile, in a small bowl stir together mustard, oil, soy sauce, and sugar substitute. Remove chicken from oven. Generously brush mustard mixture over chicken. Return to oven and continue baking for 25 minutes or until chicken is tender and no longer pink. Baste occasionally with mustard mixture. Serve warm topped with sauce from baking dish. **Nutrition**: Serves 6. Per serving: 259 calories, 14 grams fat (3 saturated), 409mg sodium, 4 grams carbohydrate and 29 grams protein.

Pepper-Lime Chicken

This chicken cooks quickly under the broiler and brings a Caribbean flair to the table. Try boneless, skinless chicken thighs if you prefer dark meat chicken.

Ingredients:
6 (4-ounce) chicken breast halves or thighs, boneless, skinless
1 teaspoon finely shredded lime peel
¼ cup lime juice
1 tablespoon canola oil
1 teaspoon dried thyme, crushed
1 teaspoon bottled minced garlic
salt and pepper to taste

Directions: Preheat broiler. Place chicken on the unheated rack of a broiler pan. Broil 4 to 5-inches from the heat for 10 minutes or until chicken starts to brown. Meanwhile, for glaze, in a small bowl stir together lime peel, lime juice, canola oil, thyme, garlic, salt, and pepper. Brush chicken with glaze. Turn chicken; brush with more glaze. Broil for 5 to 15-minutes more or until chicken is tender and no longer pink, brushing with the remaining glaze the final 5 minutes of broiling. **Nutrition**: Serves 6. Per serving: 242 calories, 28 grams protein, 13 grams fat, 2 grams carbohydrate.

Chicken with Cannellini Beans

Lean chicken with fiber-dense beans is a healthy and satisfying Day 5 meal that can be enjoyed in your ongoing pursuit of health after the 5 Day Pouch Test. The sun-dried tomato sprinkles can be found in the produce section of your supermarket. Serve sliced fresh tomatoes with this for a complete meal.

Ingredients:
cooking spray
4 (4-ounce) boneless skinless chicken breast halves
1 teaspoon dried rosemary
salt and pepper to taste
1 cup chicken broth, fat-free, reduced-sodium
1 (16-ounce) can cannellini beans, drained and rinsed
2 tablespoons sun-dried tomato sprinkles

Directions: Coat a 12-inch skillet with cooking spray and heat over medium heat until hot. Add chicken, and season with rosemary, salt, and pepper. Cook 6 to 8-minutes and turn, add chicken broth, cannellini beans, and sun-dried tomato sprinkles to skillet. Bring to a brisk simmer, reduce heat, cover and cook additional 6 minutes or more until done. Serve chicken and cannellini beans warm, drizzled with sauce. **Nutrition**: Serves 4. Per serving: 193 calories, 30 grams protein, 2 grams fat, 11 grams carbohydrate, 4 grams dietary fiber.

Chicken and Edible Pod Peas

The fresh crunch of quick-cooked pea pods and the refreshing lemon-pepper seasoning make this a light and healthy lunch or dinner on Day 5 and beyond. Edible pod peas are sometimes called snap peas, sugar-snap peas, or snow peas. Cooked edible-pod peas, also called sugar snap peas, contain three times as much vitamin C as green peas. Look for thin edible pods enclosing good-sized peas, fresh or frozen.

Ingredients:
cooking spray, butter flavor
2 teaspoons lemon-pepper seasoning, low or reduced sodium
4 (4-ounce) chicken breasts, boneless and skinless
¼ cup yogurt-based spread
1 (6-ounce) package sugar snap peas

Directions: Spray a 10-inch skillet with cooking spray and heat over medium-high heat. Season the chicken breasts with the lemon-pepper seasoning, and cook in the skillet, 8 to 12-minutes turning occasionally. Remove to a serving plate and tent loosely with foil to keep warm. Return skillet to heat and add yogurt based spread and sugar snap peas. Cook and stir for 4 to 5-minutes until just tender. Serve with warm chicken, spooning sauce over peas and chicken. **Nutrition**: Serves 4. Per serving: 259 calories, 35 grams protein, 8 grams fat, 5 grams carbohydrate.

Slow Cooker Garlic & Thyme Chicken Thighs

Take the guesswork out of Day 5 dinner when you throw this in the slow cooker first thing in the morning. The sweet orange and balsamic sauce gives new life to the standard boneless skinless chicken.

Ingredients:
6 (4-ounce) frozen boneless, skinless chicken thighs
1-2 tablespoons bottled minced garlic
1½ teaspoons dried thyme
salt and pepper to taste
½ cup orange juice
2 tablespoons balsamic vinegar
2 oranges, sliced

Directions: Place frozen chicken thighs in a 3½ to 4-quart slow cooker. In a small bowl whisk together the garlic, thyme, salt, pepper, orange juice, and balsamic vinegar and pour over chicken thighs. Cover and set to low-heat for 6 to 8-hours or high-heat for 2 to 4-hours. Just before serving strain juices into a 1-quart saucepan and bring to a boil to reduce liquid. Boil gently, uncovered, for about 10 minutes or until reduced to about 1 cup. Serve 1 thigh topped with 1 tablespoon sauce and orange slices. **Nutrition**: Serves 6. Per serving: 178 calories, 34 grams protein, 4 grams fat, 5 grams carbohydrate.

Everyone loves chicken Parmesan and this one will be ready when you get home from work. Cook spinach fettuccine for the family but enjoy yours without it. This makes great lunch leftovers for Day 6 and beyond.

Ingredients:
3 pounds chicken pieces, boneless and skinless
1 (14.5-ounce) can Italian style tomatoes
1 (6-ounce) can tomato paste
1 small onion, chopped
1 teaspoon dried Mrs. Dash® Italian Seasoning Blend
½ cup Parmesan cheese, grated

Directions: Place frozen chicken pieces in a 4-quart slow cooker. In a small bowl combine tomatoes, tomato paste, onion and Italian seasoning blend, and pour over chicken pieces. Cover and set to high for 2 to 4-hours or low for 4 to 6-hours. Serve warm with sauce sprinkled with Parmesan cheese. Serving is 4-ounces chicken and 1/3 cup sauce and 1 tablespoon Parmesan cheese. **Nutrition**: Per serving: 202 calories, 28 grams protein, 5 grams fat, 10 grams carbohydrate.

Turkey-Avocado-Swiss Stack

This is a take on a sandwich served at one of my favorite restaurants. The restaurant serves it on toasted marble rye bread. I have adapted it at home to simply be a high protein stack served on a plate, eaten with a fork. The richness of the avocado is a nice compliment to oven roasted turkey breast.

Ingredients:
16 ounces oven roasted turkey breast, sliced
4 teaspoons Miracle Whip® light
1 large avocado, sliced
4 (1-ounce) slices reduced-fat Swiss cheese
2 ounces sprouts
salt and pepper to taste

Directions: On each of four salad plates arrange 4-ounces of turkey breast slices. Spread each stack with 1 teaspoon of Miracle Whip® light. Arrange the avocado slices, sprouts, and Swiss cheese on top of each stack. Season with salt and pepper. Serve chilled. **Nutrition**: Serves 4. Per serving: 275 calories, 35 grams protein, 12 grams fat, 6 grams carbohydrate.

Turkey Tenderloin with Mustard Mushroom Sauce

The mustard mushroom sauce is rich and creamy which contributes to feelings of fullness and satiation. This is a company-worthy main dish.

Ingredients:
1½ tablespoons Mrs. Dash® Original Seasoning Blend
2 tablespoons flour
1 pound turkey tenderloin, cut into 1-inch cutlets
2 teaspoons olive oil
1 (8-ounce) package sliced mushrooms
3/4 cup chicken broth, reduced-sodium
1½ tablespoons coarse-grain mustard
2 tablespoons heavy cream

Directions: In a medium bowl combine 1 tablespoon of seasoning blend with the flour. Dredge the turkey cutlets with the flour mixture. Heat the olive oil in a 10-inch skillet over medium-high heat, add the turkey cutlets and cook until golden brown on both sides. Remove turkey from skillet to a rimmed plate and tent with foil to keep warm. Return skillet to heat, and add sliced mushrooms. Stir and cook until the mushrooms are tender. Pour chicken broth over mushrooms and cook, scraping brown pieces from bottom of the pan. Add the mustard and ½ tablespoon of seasoning blend to the sauce, and mix well. Add the heavy cream and cook and stir until the sauce is thick and well combined. Return turkey cutlets to pan with sauce to reheat. Serve each cutlet drizzled with sauce. **Nutrition**: Serves 4. Per serving: 272 calories, 28 grams protein, 14 grams fat, 7 grams carbohydrate.

Seared Pork Tenderloin Chops with Balsamic Sauce

Today's pork is lean and nutrient rich and a very good source of protein. If you cannot find boneless pork tenderloin chops purchase vacuum sealed pork tenderloin and slice into 1-inch thick chops.

Ingredients:
½ cup balsamic vinegar
½ cup beef broth, reduced-sodium
4 (4-ounce) pork tenderloin chops, boneless and trimmed of fat
salt and pepper to taste
1 tablespoon olive oil

Directions: Make sauce. Place balsamic vinegar and beef broth in a 1-quart saucepan and heat to a simmer over medium-high. Simmer until sauce is reduced and thickened, about 6 to 8 minutes. For Chops: season chops with salt and pepper on both sides. On stovetop, heat oil in a 10-inch skillet over medium-high heat. When oil is hot cook chops 5 to 8-minutes on each side, turning only once. Internal temperature should be 145°F. Serve each chop with 1 tablespoon of the balsamic sauce. **Nutrition**: Serves 4. Per serving: 213 calories, 25 grams protein, 10 grams fat, 5 grams carbohydrate.

Skillet Pork Chops with Honey-Mustard Sauce

The pork here is served with spinach, which adds fiber and nutrients to the meal, yet it remains low in carbohydrates and high in protein. Using pre-marinated pork tenderloin makes preparation swift and easy.

Ingredients:
1 (1½ pound) honey-mustard marinated pork tenderloin
pepper to taste
cooking spray
3 tablespoons lemon juice
4 green onions, finely chopped
1 (16-ounce) package frozen leaf spinach, thawed and squeezed dry

Directions: Cut the tenderloin into six equal slices and season each slice with pepper to taste. Heat a 12-inch skillet sprayed with cooking spray over medium-high heat until hot. Add pork and cook, 4 to 6 minutes per side or until done. Remove pork to a rimmed plate and tent loosely with foil. Add lemon juice and green onions to skillet and cook and stir until onions are tender. Stir in spinach, and cook, stirring constantly for 2 to 3-minutes. Divide spinach mixture among six serving plates and top each with 1 slice of pork tenderloin. **Nutrition**: Serves 6. Per serving: 166 calories, 23 grams protein, 5 grams fat, 5 grams carbohydrate.

Sirloin Steaks with Horseradish Sauce

Horseradish is a classic condiment with beef. The sour cream mixture tames the bite of this pungently spicy root. Beef sirloin is an iron-rich protein source that is also rich in vitamin B12 and zinc.

Ingredients:
1 pound sirloin steak, boneless, trimmed of excess fat
2 cloves garlic, cut in half
cooking spray
salt and pepper to taste

Sauce Ingredients:
1 clove garlic, minced
1/3 cup sour cream, fat-free
1½ tablespoons mayonnaise, reduced-fat
1 tablespoon prepared white horseradish
salt and pepper to taste

Directions: Cut steak into four (4-ounce) pieces. Rub both sides of each steak with the cut garlic. Coat a 12-inch skillet with cooking spray and place over high heat until hot. Add steaks; cook 4 minutes. Turn steaks and cook 3 minutes longer so they have a good sear. Reduce heat to medium and cook to desired doneness. Season with salt and pepper to taste. For sauce, in a small bowl combine minced garlic, sour cream, mayonnaise, prepared white horseradish, salt, and pepper. Stir well and allow to rest at room temperature until serving. **Nutrition**: Serves 4 (1 steak and 2 tablespoons sauce). Per serving: 218 calories, 27 grams protein, 9 grams fat, 5 grams carbohydrate.

Florentine T-Bone Steak

I like to use T-bone steak for this recipe but any fat-marbled thick-cut of beef will work nicely. Plan ahead as the marinating time is quite long and essential for the best results. One large steak serves four.

Ingredients:
1 (16-ounce) T-bone steak
8 tablespoons extra virgin olive oil
4-5 fresh rosemary sprigs
3 cloves garlic, crushed
sea salt and freshly ground black pepper, to taste
balsamic vinegar and olive oil, to taste

Directions: Place the steak in a shallow dish. Mix together the olive oil, rosemary, garlic, salt, and pepper. Pour over the steak, cover and marinate in the refrigerator for 24 to 48-hours turning occasionally. Remove steak from refrigerator 30 minutes prior to cooking. Heat grill or broiler to high heat. Grill the meat over direct heat turning occasionally until desired doneness. Remove from grill and allow to rest 6 to 10-minutes. Drizzle steak with balsamic vinegar and olive oil. Slice steak crosswise in thin strips to serve. **Nutrition**: One 3-ounce serving of beef T-bone steak has 161 calories, 22 grams protein, 7 grams fat.

Roasted red peppers bring a smoky flavor to this meal. Peppers are a super source of vitamin C and contain flavonoids that are believed to fight cancer. The sauce brings just enough moisture to the meat to aid chewing and digestion without it becoming a slider food.

Ingredients:
4 (4-ounce) lean beef tenderloin steaks, boneless
1 tablespoon steak seasoning
salt to taste
1 teaspoon olive oil
1 (7-ounce) jar roasted red peppers in water, drained

Directions: Season each steak with steak seasoning and salt to taste. Heat the olive oil in a 10-inch skillet over medium-high heat. When hot cook steaks 4 to 6-minutes per side. While steaks cook, place the roasted red peppers in a blender or food processor and blend until smooth. Season the sauce with salt and pepper to taste. Serve warm steaks with a drizzle of the red pepper sauce. **Nutrition**: Serves 4. Per serving: 188 calories, 25 grams protein, 3 grams carbohydrate.

Basics for Handling Food Safely

Provided by United States Department of Agriculture
Food Safety & Inspection Service
http://www.usda.gov/wps/portal/usdahome

Safe steps in food handling, cooking, and storage are essential to prevent food borne illness. You can't see, smell, or taste harmful bacteria that may cause illness

Cleanliness — Wash hands and surfaces often.
Separate — Do not cross-contaminate.
Cook — Cook to proper temperatures.
Chill — Refrigerate promptly.

Shopping
Purchase refrigerated or frozen items after selecting your non-perishables.

Never choose meat or poultry in packaging that is torn or leaking.

Do not buy food past "Sell-By," "Use-By," or other expiration dates.

Storage
Always refrigerate perishable food within 2 hours (1 hour when the temperature is above 90 °F).

Check the temperature of your refrigerator and freezer with an appliance thermometer. The refrigerator should be at 40 °F or below and the freezer at 0 °F or below.

Cook or freeze fresh poultry, fish, ground meats, and variety meats within 2 days; other beef, veal, lamb, or pork, within 3 to 5 days.

Perishable food such as meat and poultry should be wrapped securely to maintain quality and to prevent meat juices from getting onto other food.

To maintain quality when freezing meat and poultry in its original package, wrap the package again with foil or plastic wrap that is recommended for the freezer.

In general, high-acid canned food such as tomatoes, grapefruit, and pineapple can be stored on the shelf for 12 to 18 months. Low-acid canned food such as meat, poultry, fish, and most vegetables will keep 2 to 5 years — if the can remains in good condition and has been stored in a cool, clean, and dry place. Discard cans that are dented, leaking, bulging, or rusted.

Preparation
Always wash hands with warm water and soap for 20 seconds before and after handling food.

Don't cross-contaminate. Keep raw meat, poultry, fish, and their juices away from other food. After cutting raw meats, wash cutting board, utensils, and countertops with hot, soapy water.

Cutting boards, utensils, and countertops can be sanitized by using a solution of 1 tablespoon of unscented, liquid chlorine bleach in 1 gallon of water.

Marinate meat and poultry in a covered dish in the refrigerator.

Thawing
Refrigerator: The refrigerator allows slow, safe thawing. Make sure thawing meat and poultry juices do not drip onto other food.

Cold Water: For faster thawing, place food in a leak-proof plastic bag. Submerge in cold tap water. Change the water every 30 minutes. Cook Immediately after thawing.

Microwave: Cook meat and poultry immediately after microwave thawing.

Cooking
Beef, veal, and lamb steaks, roasts, and chops may be cooked to 145°F.

All uncured cuts of pork, 145°F. Cured pork should be cooked following label instructions.

Ground beef, veal and lamb to 160°F.

All poultry should reach a safe minimum internal temperature of 165°F.

Serving
Hot food should be held at 140°F or warmer.

Cold food should be held at 40°F or colder.

When serving food at a buffet, keep food hot with chafing dishes, slow cookers, and warming trays. Keep food cold by nesting dishes in bowls of ice or use small serving trays and replace them often.

Perishable food should not be left out more than 2 hours at room temperature (1 hour when the temperature is above 90 °F).

Leftovers
Discard any food left out at room temperature for more than 2 hours (1 hour if the temperature was above 90 °F).

Place food into shallow containers and immediately put in the refrigerator or freezer for rapid cooling.

Use cooked leftovers that have been properly stored within 4 days.

Bibliography

Agatston, Arthur MD. The South Beach Diet: A Doctor's Plan for Fast and Lasting Weight Loss. Headline Book Publishing, London.

Agatston, Arthur MD. The South Beach Diet: Dining Guide.Rodale, Birmingham, AL.

Bailey, Kaye (Editor). A Collection of Neighborhood Recipes: LivingAfterWLS a safe haven circle of friends. Morris Press Cookbooks, Kearney, NE.

Bailey, Kaye. Day 6: Beyond the 5 Day Pouch Test. LivingAfterWLS, LLC. Morris Printing, Kearney, NE.

Baker, Dan PhD., Stauth, Cameron. What Happy People Know. Rodale, United States.

Beard, Lina and Beard, Adelia Belle, The Original Girl's Handy Book. Black Dog & Leventhal Publishers Inc., New York, NY

Better Homes & Gardens. 15 Minutes or Less Low-Carb Recipes. Meridith Books, Des Moines, Iowa.

Better Homes & Gardens. The Smart Diet: The right approach to weight loss. Meridith Books, Des Moines, Iowa.

Brand-Miller, Jennie MD, Wolever, Thomas M.S. MD, Foster-Powell, Kaye, Colagiuri, Stephen, MD. The New Glucose Revolution: The Authoritative Guide to The Glycemic Index - the Dietary Solution for Lifelong Health. Marlowe & Company, New York, NY.

Breathnach, Sarah Ban, The Simple Abundance Companion. Warner Books, New York, NY.

Cooking Light, 5 Ingredient, 15 Minute Cookbook. Oxmoor House, Birmingham, AL.

Cooking Light, Superfast Suppers: Speedy Solutions for Dinner Dilemmas. Oxmoor House, Birmingham, AL.

Culpepper, Mary Kay (Editor). Cooking Light Magazine. Birmingham, AL.

Dayyeh, Barham K. Abu, M. D. (2011, March). Gastrojejunal Stoma Diameter Predicts Weight Regain after Roux-en-Y Gastric Bypass. Clinical Gastroenterology and Hepatology, 228-233.

Eades, Michael R. MD, Eades, Mary Dan MD. Protein Power: The High-Protein/Low-Carbohydrate Way to Lose Weight, Feel Fit, and Boost Your Health - in Just Weeks! Bantam Books, New York, NY.

Havala, Suzanne M.S., R.D. Being Vegetarian for Dummies. Wiley Publishing, Nic. Hoboken, NJ.

Institute of Medicine. (2010). Strategies to Reduce Sodium Intake in the United States. College Park, MD: FDA.

Jensen, Bernard MD. Guide to Body Chemistry & Nurtirion. Keats Publishing, Los Angeles, CA.

Johnson, Kristina M. (Editor-in-Chief). Women's Health. Rodale, Emmaus, PA.

Ketcham, Katherine, Asbury, William F. Beyond the Influence: Understanding and Defeating Alcoholism. Bantom Book. United States.

Latona, Valerie (Editor In Chief). Shape Magazine. United States.

Litin, Scott C. MD (Editor in Chief). Mayo Clinic Family Health Book. HarperResource, New York, NY.

Marber, Ian and Edgson, Vicki; The Food Doctor: Healing foods for mind and body. Collins & Brown Ltd., London.

Martha Stewart's Hors D'Oeuvres Handbook. Clarkson Potter, New York.

Mechanick, Jeffrey I. M. F. (2008, April). Medical guidelines for clinical practice for the perioperative nutritional, metabolic, and nonsurgical support of the bariatric surgery patient. Endocrine Practice, 318-336.

Natow, Annette B.; Heslin PhD., RD, Jo-Ann M.A., R.D. The Protein Counter, 2nd Edition. Pocket Books, New York, NY.

Ostman, Barbara Gibbs; Baker, Jane L. The Recipe Writer's Handbook. John Wiley & Sons, Inc., Hoboken, NJ.

Reader's Digest, Eat Well Stay Well. Reader's Digest Association, Inc. Pleasantville, NY.

Rewega, Alicia (Editor). Clean Eating. Mississauga, Ontario, Canada.

Rohaiem, Anne E. E. (2011). Prevention Best Weight Loss Recipes. New York: Rodale Inc.

Smith, Art. Back to the Table; The Reunion of Food and Family. Hyperion: New York. 2001.

Swilley, Dana RD. UCLA Division of General Surgery, Section of Minimally Invasive and Bariatric Surgery. "Micronutrient and Macronutrient Needs in Roux-en-Y Gastric Bypass Patients. March 2008. Bariatric Times.

The Best of Gourmet, 20th Anniversary Edition. Conde' Nast Books, Random House, New York.

The New Mayo Clinic Cookbook, Eating Well for Better Health. Oxmoor House, Birmingham, AL.

Turner, Elizabeth (Editor in Chief). Vegetarian Times. El Segundo, CA.

Weil, Andrew MD, Daley, Rosie. The Healthy Kitchen, Recipes for a Better Body, Life, and Spirit. Alfred A. Knopf, New York, NY.

Whitney, Ellie, Rolfes, Sharon Rady. Understanding Nutrition. Thomson & Wadsworth. United States.

Wittgrove, A. C. (1999). Discharge Instructions for Gastric Bypass. San Diego: Alvarado Center for Surgical Weight Control.

Wurtman, Judith JP., & Nina Frusztajer Marquis, M. (2006). The Serotonin Power Diet. New York City: Rodale.

Overview of Metabolic & Bariatric Surgery

by American Society for Metabolic and Bariatric Surgery (2008)
I provide this report, without editing or interpretation, for your reference.

Overview:

Treatment for morbid obesity and obesity-related diseases and condition; limits amount of food stomach can hold, and/or limits amount of calories absorbed, by surgically reducing the stomach's capacity to a few ounces.

Candidates have a body mass index (BMI) of 40 or more, or a BMI of 35 or more with an obesity-related disease, such as Type 2 diabetes, heart disease or sleep apnea.

About 220,000 people with morbid obesity in the U.S. had bariatric surgery in 2008

About 15 million people in the U.S. have morbid obesity; 1% of the clinically eligible population is being treated for morbid obesity through bariatric surgery.

Bariatric surgery costs an average of $17,000 - $26,000; insurance coverage varies by provider.

Impact on Obesity-Related Diseases:

Can improve or resolve more than 30 obesity-related conditions, including Type 2 diabetes, heart disease, sleep apnea, hypertension and high cholesterol.

Gastric bypass resolves Type 2 diabetes in nearly 87% of patients.

Band surgery resolves Type 2 diabetes in 73% of patients.

Cuts risk of developing coronary heart disease in half.

Resolves obstructive sleep apnea in more than 85% of patients.

Bariatric Surgery: Risks vs. Benefits:

In 2007, Federal government (Agency for Healthcare Research and Quality) and clinical studies report significant improvements in safety.

Risk of death from bariatric surgery is about 0.1%.

Bariatric surgery increases lifespan, as compared to those who do not have surgery.

Patients may improve life expectancy by 89%.

Patients may reduce their risk of premature death by 30 to 40%.

Dramatic reduction in risk of death from obesity-related diseases, as compared to those who do not have surgery.

Risk of death from diabetes down 92%, from cancer down 60% and from coronary artery disease down 56%.

Long-Term Effectiveness of Bariatric Surgery:

Typically patients have maximum weight loss within 1-2 years after surgery and maintain a substantial weight loss, with improvements in obesity-related conditions, for years afterwards.

Patients may lose 30 to 50% of their excess weight 6 months after surgery and 77% of their excess weight as early as 12 months after surgery.

Long-term studies show up to 10-14 years after surgery, morbidly obese patients who had surgery maintained a much greater weight loss and more favorable levels of diabetes, cholesterol and hypertension, as compared to those who did not have surgery.

Adolescents and Bariatric Surgery:

As obesity rates rise in the U.S., increasing number of adolescents (12-17 years old) are having bariatric surgery; an estimated 349 in 2004

Research shows that bariatric surgery may be an effective treatment for Type 2 diabetes, high blood pressure and high cholesterol in extremely obese adolescents

Long-term efficacy and impact is subject of ongoing research

Most Common Types of Bariatric Surgery:

Gastric Bypass: Stomach reduced from size of football to size of golf ball. Smaller stomach is attached to middle of small intestine, bypassing the section of the small intestine (duodenum) that absorbs the most calories. Patients eat less because stomach is smaller and absorb fewer calories because food does not travel through duodenum.

Laparoscopic Adjustable Gastric Banding (LAGB): Silicone band filled with saline is wrapped around upper part of stomach to create small pouch and cause restriction. Patients eat less because they feel full quickly. Size of restriction can be adjusted after surgery by adding or removing saline from band.

Bilio-Pancreatic Diversion with Duodenal Switch: Similar to gastric bypass, but surgeon creates sleeve-shaped stomach. Smaller stomach is attached to final section of small intestine, bypassing the duodenum. Patients eat less because the stomach is smaller and absorb fewer calories because food does not travel through the duodenum.

Newer Procedures & Surgical Devices:

Vertical Sleeve Gastrectomy: Stomach restricted by stapling and dividing it vertically, removing more than 85%. Procedure generates weight loss by restricting the amount of food that can be eaten. Currently indicated as an alternative to gastric banding

Natural Orifice Translumenal Endoscopic Surgery (NOTES): Emerging minimally invasive procedure still in clinical trials. Surgery performed through natural orifice such as mouth or vagina, eliminating need for external incisions. Patients may experience a quicker, less painful recovery.

Source: American Society for Metabolic and Bariatric Surgery
Contact: Keith Taylor (212) 527-7537
http://www.asmbs.org

Day ___ Journal

Notes:

Records:	Nutritional Intake – All food and Beverages				
Day/Date: Weight:	Item	Pro(g)	Fat(g)	Carbs(g)	Calories
Water Goal: 0 0 0 0 0 0 0 0 0 0 Mark 1 bubble for each 8-ounce serving water.					
Vitamins/Supplements:					
Exercise & Fitness:					
Goals/ Totals:					

Summary:

Day ___ Journal

Notes:

Records:	Nutritional Intake – All food and Beverages				
Day/Date: Weight:	Item	Pro(g)	Fat(g)	Carbs(g)	Calories
Water Goal: 0 0 0 0 0 0 0 0 0 0 Mark 1 bubble for each 8-ounce serving water.					
Vitamins/Supplements:					
Exercise & Fitness:					
Goals/ Totals:					

Summary:

Index

Kaye Bailey developed the 5 Day Pouch Test in 2007 and is the owner of LivingAfterWLS and the 5 Day Pouch Test websites. Ms. Bailey, a professional research journalist, and a bariatric RNY (gastric bypass) patient since 1999, brings professional research methodology and personal experience to her publications focused on long-lasting successful weight management after surgery.

Concerned about weight regain her bariatric surgeon advised her to "get back to basics". With that vague advice Ms. Bailey says, "I read thousands of pages and conducted interviews with medical professionals including surgeons, nutritionists, and mental health providers. I collected data from WLS post-ops who honestly and generously shared their experience. My research background gave me the methodology to collect a vast amount of data. As a patient I found answers to the questions and concerns I have in common with most patients after WLS." From that the 5DPT and related works evolved.

Kaye Bailey is the author of countless articles syndicated in several languages, and books available in print and electronic format including The 5 Day Pouch Test Owner's Manual; Day 6: Beyond the 5 Day Pouch Test; Cooking with Kaye Methods to Meals: Protein First Recipes You Will Love.

The LivingAfterWLS Neighborhood

Sunset Announcement October 2013: The LivingAfterWLS Neighborhood proudly served the international weight loss community from 2006 through 2013 providing a safe haven meeting place of support and kindness for fellow weight loss surgery patients. It is with mixed feelings we say *Goodbye* as the sun sets on our Neighborhood.

The constantly changing and increasing technologic demands required to keep a community of this size operational and secure are too much for our small company to bear. Our resources are better spent providing quality, well-researched content via our other media channels and print publications.

As we close the gates we thank the membership, thousands of stellar individuals who selflessly supported one another in a fine example that we are not ever alone in this weight loss surgery experience.

Day 6: Beyond the 5 Day Pouch Test – 2nd Printing
By Kaye Bailey © 2009, 2012
Kaye Bailey's bestselling book: Day 6: Beyond the 5 Day Pouch Test. You've succeeded with the 5 Day Pouch Test. Keep the momentum by learning the secrets of Day 6 - Beyond the 5 Day Pouch Test. Facts, Inspiration, Recipes all in Kaye's empowering style. Sixty-six new recipes, 220 pages, soft cover book: recommended by bariatric centers everywhere. Save $4.00 off publisher price! Available at the LivingAfterWLS General Store: $25.95

Cooking with Kaye: Methods to Meals
Protein First Recipes You Will Love
by Kaye Bailey (C) 2012
134 Irresistible Recipes - Tips & Hints - Nutritional Wisdom

Kaye Bailey's all-new highly anticipated cookbook is a hit in the WLS community. Written for the weight loss surgery patient and the people they cook for, this hard-back comb bound cookbook features 134 all new recipes and detailed techniques to take you beyond the meal to create recipes you and your family will love. Recipe categories include soups, salads, crunchy protein, savory skillet meals, oven baking and roasting, braising and slow cooking. Enjoy something delicious today: get Cooking with Kaye. Cooking with Kaye is suitable for all bariatric procedures including gastric bypass, adjustable gastric banding, gastric sleeve and others. Available at the LivingAfterWLS General Store: $23.95

Websites:

LivingAfterWLS.com

5DayPouchTest.com

LAWLSBookstore.com

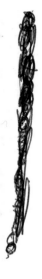

Made in the USA
Lexington, KY
06 April 2017